Nurse Mary

Nurse Mary

The Recollections of a Nurse during the American
Civil War & Franco-Prussian War

Adventures of an Army Nurse in Two Wars,

Mary Phinney, Baroness von Olnhausen

James Phinney Munroe

With a Short Biographical Account of the
Superintendent of Nurses Dorothea L. Dix
by L. P. Brockett

LEONAUR

Nurse Mary
The Recollections of a Nurse during the American Civil War & Franco-Prussian War
Adventures of an Army Nurse in Two Wars, Mary Phinney, Baroness von Olnhausen
by James Phinney Munroe
With a Short Biographical Account of the Superintendent of Nurses Dorothea L. Dix
by L. P. Brockett

FIRST EDITION

Leonaur is an imprint of Oakpast Ltd

Copyright in this form © 2017 Oakpast Ltd

ISBN: 978-1-78282-674-3 (hardcover)
ISBN: 978-1-78282-675-0 (softcover)

http://www.leonaur.com

Publisher's Notes

Contents

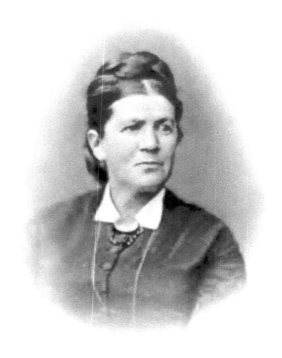

Mary von Othkausen.

Chapter 1

In the south part of the historic town of Lexington, Massachusetts, lies a farm of many acres gently sloping from high, wooded hills on the east towards the valley of Hobbs Brook now converted into a reservoir for Cambridge on the west. Divided by the shaded country road which leads from Lexington village, past the birthplace of Theodore Parker, to the city of Waltham, this farm comprises on the one side orchards and cultivated meadows, on the other a wide expanse of grassland sweeping in soft curves around the site of the dwelling-house and accented at the roadway's edge by magnificent rock maples brought from New Hampshire by "Squire" Phinney seventy years ago. This estate, the beauty of which is unsurpassed in Lexington, was almost continuously, from 1786 to 1849, the home of Elias Phinney, the father of Mary (Phinney) von Olnhausen.

The first New England Phinney, John, came to Cape Cod about nine years after the landing of the Pilgrims, and settled in what is now the town of Scituate. His son John married Mary Rogers, granddaughter to that Thomas Rogers who was a passenger on the first *Mayflower* voyage and a signer of the "Compact." In the third generation from them was a Benjamin Phinney who, since he removed to Granville, Nova Scotia, in 1774, and did not return until 1786, it is fair to presume was a Tory. This suspicion is deepened by the fact that he did not come back to Falmouth, where he was born, but to Lexington, at that time remote enough from Cape Cod to escape any possible lingerings of local animosity.

This Benjamin Phinney and his wife, Susanna, had nine children. Of these the seventh, and the last to be born in Nova Scotia, was Elias, who, at the age of six, came with his father and mother to the farm in Lexington. Educated in the district school and by the harder tuition of a large farm; practised, too, in cabinet making, which was his father's trade, Elias fitted himself for Harvard College, paid his own way there, and was graduated in the Class of 1801. Electing thereafter to follow the law, he studied with an eminent lawyer in Maine and practised his profession in Thomaston for about ten years.

Eight years after his graduation from Harvard, Elias Phinney married Catherine Bartlett, daughter of Dr. Josiah Bartlett, of Charlestown, Massachusetts. This Dr. Bartlett, born in 1759, had attended Harvard College. His studies interrupted by the opening Revolution, he had taken up surgery in the office of Dr. Isaac Foster, and, as surgeon's mate, had tended the wounded of Bunker Hill and of later battles of the War for Independence. Not only in surgery, but in history and archaeology, Dr. Bartlett made for himself an honoured name; and, as a Mason, he repeatedly filled the office of Grand Warden of the Grand Lodge of Massachusetts. A funeral oration upon George Washington, an address of welcome to President Monroe when that official visited Charlestown, and a history of Charlestown are among the literary productions of a man who was a leading citizen of his day and town. Dr. Bartlett married Elizabeth Call, of Charlestown, and by her had sixteen children, of whom the second, Catherine, became the wife of Elias Phinney.

Two or three years after their marriage, the Phinneys removed from Thomaston to Charlestown, and he continued there the practice of the law, holding many estates in trust, and taking a prominent part in the affairs of the town until, in 1823, his father being then over seventy years of age and unable to carry on the work of the farm alone, Elias, who had always hungered for agriculture, was easily persuaded to return to Lexington. After removing to that town, he continued to go daily to his office in Charlestown, there to carry on an ever-increasing practice of the law, until in 1831 he was appointed Clerk of the Judicial Court for the County of Middlesex. He entered upon his duties June 19, 1831, and from that time until his death faithfully attended the sittings during the sessions of the court and went daily to the Court House in East Cambridge in vacations.

Only on Thursdays of those vacations was he free to stay at home; and it is extra ordinary that with such limited opportunity for supervision, with regular duties which often took him from Lexington before daylight and kept him away until after dark, he could have accomplished so much in agriculture.

For, in a day when scientific methods were almost unknown, scientific agriculture became increasingly Mr. Phinney's avocation. He was for many years a trustee of the State Agricultural Society; he was active in the importation and breeding of Ayrshire cattle; new fruits and vegetables, including the tomato, were the subject of his ceaseless experimentation; while the genuine study of fertilizers, of soils, of rotation of crops, of breeding, of grafting, gave him a wide reputation among those to whom farming meant something more than a routine of ploughing, sowing, and reaping. This widely known experimentation, his seven charming daughters (Harvard College was but five miles away), and his abundant hospitality made his house a centre for learned and brilliant men, both old and young. "No man in Massachusetts," it is declared in a sketch of him, "had so large a circle of friends;" and this statement, in various phrasing, is the keynote of every notice which his death called forth. Chief-Justice Shaw, Josiah Quincy, Dr. Warren, Daniel Webster, Rufus Choate, the Lawrences, were but a few of the host of those who sought and always found a welcome at his house.

His vocation, the law, and his avocation, farming, still left him time to take active part in the affairs of Lexington. His name was for many years prominent in the annals of the town; it was he who welcomed Lafayette when that remarkable man came to Lexington; it was he who presided when, in April, 1835, the bodies of those who had been killed at the Battle of Lexington were removed from the old cemetery to their present resting-place and Edward Everett made his famous oration; it was he who, as chairman of a committee appointed by the town, took the affidavits of the survivors of the battle, and with those as a basis wrote an authentic and graphic history of that memorable day.

Of a commanding though always courteous bearing, a man of the world and yet intensely devoted to the interests of his adopted town, the enlightened possessor and developer of many fruitful acres, the dispenser of a hospitality as simple as it was unbounded, Elias Phinney early secured and always retained the rather unusual title of "Squire." To an extraordinary degree he fulfilled the English idea of that title, glorifying it, moreover, with the higher ideals of his American environment.

In the summer of 1847 there fell upon him a blow of peculiar sadness. The house in which, with the exception of a few years, he had lived for six decades was destroyed by fire, together with the greater portion of its contents and many of the fine shade-trees which he had taken so much pleasure in planting. Within a few days, however, over three thousand dollars to build another house had been subscribed and sent to him, with warmest expressions of sympathy and regard. Chief among these liberal givers were the Lawrences, Peter C. Brooks, David Sears, John C. Gray, Dr. Warren, John Welles, Henry Codman, Francis C. Lowell, William P. Mason, Josiah Quincy, and James Vila.

He did not, however, long survive. Hardly had the family moved into their new home, scarcely had he begun to try to repair the ravages of the flames on his beloved shade-trees, when, on the 24th of July, 1849, Mr. Phinney died in the sixty-ninth year of his age. His widow survived him fourteen years.

Elias and Catherine Phinney had ten children,—seven daughters and three sons. The fifth child and the fourth daughter was Mary, born on the third day of February, 1818. Receiving her earlier schooling at the Franklin—familiarly known as the "Kite End"—district school, Mary later attended the Lexington Academy, and finally was a pupil at Smith's Academy in Waltham. Both these schools had local reputation; and the building occupied by the Lexington Academy was later made famous by the fact that there, in 1839, was established, under the mastership of Cyrus Peirce, the first Normal School in the United States.

Living an active life on a busy and extensive farm, performing necessarily a large share of the labour of the house and the garden, the daughters of the Phinney household were not infected by the fashion of that time requiring young women to be languishing, pearly-hued, timid, accomplished only in "ladylike" but wholly useless arts. Rather they seem to have anticipated the young women of the present day; for they were active, unaffected, healthy, vigorous, able to turn their hands to any sort of useful labour. Mary, however, was more "emancipated" even than the others. Some years before the day of Mrs. Bloomer, she fashioned for herself out of calico a "bloomer" costume which she wore when at work in the garden.

At a time when to be ignorant of nature was thought a sign of good breeding, she knew every flower and insect of the wood and field; in a generation whose women shuddered at a grasshopper, she used to tame spiders and to give pocket-refuge to toads and snakes; in an age whose pale heroines were occupied mainly in graceful swooning, she acted the nurse and surgeon for every wound in a populous and venturesome neighbourhood. Farm work, too, had the highest interest for her; and with perhaps a little, characteristic exaggeration she used to recall the many moonlight evenings on which she helped her father—that being his only leisure time—graft apple-trees until ten o'clock at night. An accomplished needlewoman, as were all the sisters, Mary had also a marked talent for drawing, the exercise of which was to prove the real vocation of her life.

The death of Mr. Phinney in 1849 compelled the sale of his farm, and threw those of his daughters who were yet unmarried upon their own resources. Mary, taking advantage of her unusual facility in drawing, sought employment as a designer of print goods, then an absolutely new career for women. The mills of those days were, however, quite different from the factories of today. Even the unskilled mill girl then was not in the least akin to those bold and unkempt women, mainly foreigners, who now, (1904), are seen streaming from the establishments of our great factory towns. What those mill girls were may be understood by a few extracts from Lucy Larcom's *A New England Girlhood*. She says:—

> What were we? Girls who were working in a factory for the time, to be sure; but none of us had the least idea of continuing at that kind of work permanently. Our composite photograph, had it been taken, would have been the representative New England girlhood of those days. We had all been fairly educated at public or private schools, and many of us were resolutely bent upon obtaining a better education. Very few among us were without some distinct plan for bettering the condition of themselves and those they loved.
>
> For the first time, our young women had come forth from their home retirement in a throng, each with her own individual purpose. For twenty years or so, Lowell might have been looked upon as a rather select industrial school for young people. The girls there were just such girls as are knocking at the doors of young women's colleges today. They had come to work with their hands, but they could not hinder the working of their minds also. Their mental activity was overflowing at every possible outlet. . . .
>
> I regard it as one of the privileges of my youth that I was permitted to grow up among those active, interesting girls, whose lives were not mere echoes of other lives, but had principle and purpose distinctly their own. Their vigour of character was a natural development. The New Hampshire girls who came to Lowell were descendants of the sturdy backwoods men who settled that State scarcely a hundred years before. Their grand-

11

mothers had suffered the hard ships of frontier life, had known the horrors of savage warfare when the beautiful valleys of the Connecticut and the Merrimack were threaded with Indian trails from Canada to the white settlements. Those young women did justice to their inheritance. They were earnest and capable; ready to undertake anything that was worth doing.

Employed first at Dover, New Hampshire, in the Cocheco Mills, Mary Phinney afterwards went to the Manchester Print Works, at Manchester, New Hampshire. In both cities, she made many delightful friendships that were destined to continue all her life. Especially in Manchester did she find agreeable associates among the cultivated Germans who, driven from their own country by the pressure following the political revolutions there, had sought refuge in free America, and were putting that extraordinary technical knowledge in which they have so long led the world to practical use in the rapidly developing manufactures of New England. Conspicuous in this congenial German-American colony was Gustav, Baron von Olnshausen, or, as he preferred to call himself, Gustav A. Olnhausen.

The von Olnhausen family is of that old "Freiherr" stock, to belong to which places one, in German eyes, above foreign princes and but little below their own kings. Its unquestioned history runs back for many centuries; and its old castle of Schoenfels, perched high upon the hills overlooking Zwickau, Saxony (about sixty miles from Dresden), is surrounded by a moat and is—or at least was—furnished with all the appurtenances of a mediaeval stronghold. Gustav, born about 1810, was the last male, in the direct line, of this old family. Receiving his education at that period, culminating in the revolutions of 1848, when all Germany was in political ferment, he imbibed, and doubtless advocated, democratic ideas that made it wise, if not indeed necessary, for him to live away from his native Saxony.

His history before coming to America is not definitely known, (see Appendix A); but it is certain that he resided for some years in Russia, acquiring fluent knowledge of the language of that country, and that he travelled extensively in other lands. In Germany or elsewhere he gained what for those days was an unusual proficiency in the science and art of chemistry. Theodore Parker, who knew him well, declared him to be one of the most learned men that he had ever met. Entirely out of sympathy with the feudal institutions and atmosphere of his native country, the income of his estate so reduced by changed commercial conditions as to have necessitated the sale of the old home at Zwickau, his sisters and half-sisters married, Gustav von Olnhausen came finally to America, was doubtless attracted by the other Germans living there to Manchester, New Hampshire, and found employment, as chemist, in the dye-houses of the Manchester Mills.

★★★★★★

One of his sisters married a von Roemer, and another a von Rohrscheidt. As will appear later, their brother's widow visited these ladies (themselves then widowed) after the Franco-Prussian War, spending with them and with others of her husband's relatives two of the most delightful years of her life.

★★★★★★

In that city, he met Mary Phinney, loved her, and soon found that she too loved him. Most worthy, too, of her affection he must have been. Learned in language, in literature, in science, he was nevertheless as unassuming as a little child; brought up in the formal etiquette of a German provincial town, he was as simple and unconventional as was Miss Phinney, herself a rebel against the restrictions placed about the women of her day; a member of an aristocracy that still believes in the divine right of kings and nobles, he was a democrat of the sturdiest, most thoroughgoing sort. All these qualities appealed to her as did her free, vigorous womanhood to him; and their engagement seems to have been a foregone conclusion long before it became an actual fact.

The economic value of technically trained men was, however, then so little recognised, the panic of 1857 had so hampered business and manufacturing, that Mr. von Olnhausen's salary seems to have been very small. Not until more than a year after their engagement, therefore, did he find himself financially able to marry; and, after marriage, their housekeeping was of a most modest sort. A little house filled with flowers, ferneries, aquaria (for they were alike in their love of nature), and peopled with birds, lizards, and even tamed toads, was the centre of their happiness; their chief pleasure, beyond that of their perfectly sympathetic life together, being found in their work, in holiday walks through the woods, and in picnics and little impromptu parties with their many friends.

That simple way of enjoying life which the Germans have learned and which we Americans have not, was as congenial to Mary von Olnhausen as it was to her husband; and her brief years of marriage were undoubtedly the happiest of all her life. The only interruption of their gentle tranquillity was in her occasional visits to Lexington and to Watertown, where she had relatives and friends.

A glimpse of this happy time is given in the following letters of Mr. von Olnhausen's, the first two written before their marriage, the third after that fortunate event.

Wednesday evening.

My Own Dear Molly,—Instead of the intended company, I am writing you, and I really enjoy it much better. K. is sick since a few days and so I better postponed the assembly, but anyhow I shall have it sometimes this week for celebrating the merry Christmas. I liked this feast so much as child and old remembrances let me like it now yet. I should like we could it pass sometimes in Germany—they think so much about it there—it's principally a merry time for the children, but old people enjoy it just as much. We shall pass much happier the next than this one—my dear girl—at least I, and anywhere we shall be. I shall quite arrange it in German fashion.

I remember home so often this evening, for it's the time when everyone is quite busy in the preparations—and quite happy already in its expectations—a quite pleasant evening. The ladies whirling round yet in the full pride of domestic activeness and making use of all sciences for producing delicacies and dainties, such as never are seen in the whole other part of the year; red the lively faces from excitement and kitchen-heat, they distribute a few small specimens of their artfulness, just to hear praised themselves and to be fervently asked for a few more:—the gentlemen—in the meantime are preparing the Christmas-tree, gilding nuts and apples, fixing the wax-candles and fastening threads round all the stars and candies and sugar-figures, destined for swinging between the branches of the enchanted tree. The children are already sent to bed, full of the expectation of the coming day—all have been during the last weeks the best children of the world, afraid to lose by disobedience love and presents of the little Christ and just as anxious about it as I am about your love.

What a nice present I shall give you next year my sweet child, when you have been good, and have I been so, I am sure, you will recompense me and be it only by a kiss. Are we not both like children yet—why should we not remain so our whole life? Children only, it is said, go to heaven—but also here on earth we shall not be childish but the more childrenlike the happier we are.

Piscatoquaw Valley.

My Dear Molly,—May it be made known to my queen, that I just am feeling myself in a state of mind and body, as no other king of earth can feel better—provided he is a bachelor. My throne I rest upon is glittering from mica and garnets, green moss is spread round and like a beautiful carpet widely but tastefully embroidered with mayflowers, cheering at once the eyes and the (how prosaically nose sounds) odoriferous sense. It is true the banquet, just finished, consisted only in sausage and crackers, but the appetite makes the meal and not the dishes. Just beside me a small brook offers me its cool and clear water for refreshment, and is murmuring to me so many confuse and strange stories like from the fairy land. The song of hundreds of frogs will not harmonise well with the dreams of the brook, but they are in a proper distance,—distance improves everything—and you are in my mind so near associated with them, so that I don't hear exactly your voice, your dear voice, amongst them—no—but that I really imagine I hear them call your name.

I wonder if you knew that we have Fastday today and came to take the walk with me. I cannot thank heaven enough for sending us such a beautiful day—for it should be really hard to spend such an excited day in town. My principal aim today is less natural history than walking, for I feel how much I need it after that frightful weather. But anyhow besides some bugs and beetles I got a green snake, I am very glad of for trying my alcohol substitute in respect of the change of the colour, and—an old, of course—but entirely new bird's nest entirely made from lichens, I never have seen before.

Now I am sitting between Manchester and Goffstown, where I came partly on the railroad, partly along the right bank of the Squaw R.—and can probably not be far from Goffstown. I cannot find any bridge over that little river—to go the same road back is too tiresome and probably not much shorter—*en avant*—courage then—soon more from my headquarters. (Friday morning.) The poor king of the day in what a helpless condition he came home in the evening! What a humiliating lesson for his pride! But why? Kings can be tired like other people and sooner yet. Without a strengthening glass of cider in the Amoskeag Hotel I don't know if I ever should have reached home. And then at home how delicious the tea, how savoury the boiled potatoes, and for dessert an orange—and the king was king again!

Sunday evening.

My Dear Wife,—The day passed better than I expected;—when you stay much longer, I shall quite fall back in my old bachelor's habits and faults. I staid at home till 3 p.m. in the highest enjoyment an Italian thinks life can offer, in a *dolce far niente*, just to do what you like and should it be nothing. There was quite a summer heat à *la* Molly,—and I found only a little consolation in the thought, that I am sure, you are at least comfortable, one of the "perhaps few" mortal souls who could be so in that foretaste of hell or purgatory where the Catholics think we must all come to. At 3 p.m. Mr. M. came to fetch me for a walk and we fetched O. and out we went and had a hard work through fields and woods.

We had a really first rate supper at O.'s—Dandelion's Salad and ham and potatoes and tea and sour cider. Be glad that you are not here today (Monday) for of course, I am cross like a crow. It's only 5 a.m. and I am already writing you, but of course, having neglected my duty, not to have written you yesterday, how could I have slept longer! I wonder that I could sleep at all and more so that I slept as sound as I did.

I was really unhappy Saturday night coming 2 minutes too late to the Post office, but I got your letter just now. I am mad—like—like—I don't know anything what can be so mad so there is now an ink spot on the clean table (it is yours), but what do I care. I am mad and will not write a single letter more—"*instead Wednesday you come only Thursday.*" I know, I shall see you no more this week; your next letter will add again a day more and so on. I unfortunate, stupid and most enamoured of all husbands. When my rage has subsided, perhaps tomorrow—perhaps today already, more! I will not say "stay as long as you will" for you might really be capable to stay till to the world's end. When you love me you come soon.

Mad! That . . . cider and your letter—you shall not have an aquarium, you don't deserve it, you don't love me; but anyhow

I will be true and will love you as I have done from now till in all eternity, Amen. You see, better feelings overcome already my madness; but I will not be good today, and I shall let whither all the fine bouquets I have decorated the room with, and shoot the blinds and let not light and sun in and go to bed—no—to work. Do the same and be a good girl (perhaps anyhow I build you an aquarium) and remember and love your loving

Gustav.

They were married on May Day, 1858, by Theodore Parker. Within little more than two years, Mr. von Olnhausen developed a serious organic disease from which relief had finally to be sought through a surgical operation. (See Appendix B.) For this he went to the Massachusetts General Hospital in Boston. The operation was successful; but, other complications arising, it was impossible for the patient to rally; and he died after several weeks of pain, borne with much fortitude, on the seventh of September, 1860.

To remain single until one's fortieth year; then to love and to be loved with the ardour and simplicity of youth; and, in the third year of marriage, to lose one's husband was, of course, a crucial experience. It might have made a less active and unselfish nature hard, brooding, hopeless, and embittered. With Mary von Olnhausen, this tremendous experience proved to be really the beginning of her life. That love which might have been given, had he lived, solely to her husband, was to be expended during the coming years for others; that activity which might have been limited to the little house in Manchester was to find conspicuous satisfaction on both sides of the world.

Chapter 2

Within two months after the death of Mr. von Olnhausen, his widow had determined to begin her work for others by going to the help of her younger brother and his invalid wife, in Illinois. This brother, George, as enamoured as was his father of agriculture, had been tempted by the wonderful fertility of the middle West to leave the rocky hillsides of New England for those vast prairies whose virgin soil was as rich as it was easy of cultivation. The life of the pioneer, however, is never comfortable; limited capital and remoteness from markets made the working of the Illinois farmland unusually difficult and uncertain; drought and destructive insects often played havoc with the crops; and, worst of all, the hard life and the malarial atmosphere distressingly, and at last fatally, affected the wife's health.

With four little children, and with their mother almost incapacitated by hardship and by ague, the brother was certainly in great need of such help as his sister Mary could give; and she did not hesitate to take what was then a serious journey, and to place herself in conditions which she knew to be both difficult and disagreeable. In the following extracts from that autobiography, which, at the earnest wish of her friends, she began several years before her death, she gives a vivid impression of her arrival on the prairie, and of some of the incidents of her life there.

(FROM THE *AUTOBIOGRAPHY*.)

A six hours ride over the prairie with just enough snow to limit the landscape and not enough to hide the deep black mud which seemed to swallow the struggling oxen and horses, made one glad that the next station was the end of this tiresome journey. I did not know what desolation was until I came in sight of that station,—a barn-like structure, with one single house as companion, planted in the everlasting mud. I could not believe it was the right place, especially as no carriage was waiting and no soul was visible but the station-master, who led me into a barren room and bade me sit until my brother should appear. The windows were curtained with dust, the fire nearly out, and the chair hard and uncomfortable. After a dreary wait, a wagon came in sight,—a long, low wagon without springs drawn by a sorry pair of mules, the driver sitting in a rush-bottomed chair. This proved to be my brother and the expected "carriage." After shaking off the snow and greeting me warmly, he put the trunks on the wagon, sat on one of them, and gave me the chair. Starting off at the slowest imaginable pace, I soon made acquaintance with a slough, a ditch of mud, that might sometime have been a bottom less stream, so wide and deep that it seemed impossible ever to reach the other side. Not a house was in sight,—and indeed one could not see, the snow became so thick, and we rode and rode as if it would never end. The great sorrow I had left behind came back with twofold force, and the desolation of that dismal prairie hidden by falling snow was more than I could bear.

At last we came to a little house standing upon four posts, with free play for the winds beneath. At its open door were clustered three or four children eagerly looking for the new friend. But how to get to those expectant faces, with just a very slanting board leading up to them? Outstretched hands, however, helped me up the slippery plank, a warm welcome and a cup of hot tea soon comforted one, and the children were pretty and good; so, I became able to answer eager questions and to talk of the delicious things in store for them in the morning, when the boxes and trunks should be opened. I had so much to relate that it was late when we went to bed, which involved taking a now sleeping child under one's arm, scrambling up a ladder, and crawling through a hole into the only other room of the house. In this attic-room, with only a quilt dividing it, all the household, except the hired man, slept.

The morning waking was cold and forlorn enough; the house being neither plastered nor shingled, every breath of wind swept through it. The well had been dry for weeks, so all had to be set at work to melt snow. The wife was too feeble, from a long "spell" of chills, to do any work, so it all fell to me, and it seemed like one of those tasks set by cruel masters in fairy books. A grand dinner was improvised for the day, but the morrow was to be the sacred feast of Thanksgiving. I had timed my visit for this special occasion. As soon as we had dined, the boy, six years old, was put upon one of the mules, and was sent, with true Western hospitality, to invite the only neighbours with whom they "visited" to the coming feast, and we all began the preparations. The pudding and pies were all from home and had only to be heated; but that turkey was of wonderful size and needed much work to make it ready for the oven.

The next morning was sunny and delightful. At ten o'clock the neighbour's wagon appeared,—a wagon with springs and drawn by quite swift horses. It was considered a wonderful turnout. This neighbour's family consisted of father, mother, two boys, and the wife's brother; they were people who had lived in a town, knew what good things were, and proved pleasant and intelligent. The men, in Western fashion, sat with chairs tipped back against the wall, the children rushed up and down the ladder, making all the noise they could, so one can imagine what that room was with seven grown people and six children and the mud and steam and odours from the stove. But to see the enjoyment of them all when the dinner was served was a real pleasure. This was an unheard-of day on the prairie and was long talked of.

When the spring began to come all was changed; the wonderful sounds were enchanting and so new to me. The wild geese and ducks passing overhead from morning till night, the crows trumpeting, the prairie chickens calling their mates, and the variety of beautiful flowers,—all made the prairie seem like paradise. One could see seven miles, both east and west, to where the "timber" grew, and only three houses in all that wide extent.

One morning, just as we were breakfasting with some friends who had come to pass the night, a man rode up to the door in great haste, saying, "Mr. Phinney, what ails your corn-patch?"

"Nothing, only that I have the best stand of corn in the country."

"Well, go look at it now."

My brother went out without hat or breakfast, for it was a long distance to the corn-patch, and we went up to the chamber window. The whole land as far as we could see was bare,—not a green thing. Then, of course, we rushed out, and such a sight! The ground was covered with a moving mass of worms several inches deep, one layer crawling over another. George said it was the army worm, of which there was some tradition, though no one had ever seen it there. George rushed, got the mules out, and ploughed a deep trench at the edge of the field, for they were making for his wheat field. Then he fastened a log to a horse and all day long a boy rode back and forth crushing the worms as they fell into the ditch. For a few hours in the night they stopped;

but at break of day they started again and the log was once more put in motion. By this means the wheat and vegetables were saved. I shall never forget the discouragement on George's face as he saw all his spring work destroyed and with it his hopes of paying for his farm.

My cousin, Dr. B., who was staying with us, said to me, "Will you help me plant it over?" Of course, I was glad to do anything; so though George said it was no use, fresh corn was shelled and the old corn-planter put in order. This was a very clumsy affair, one of the earliest made. It had a button on the wheels, and whenever that turned up a lever was pulled out, and the corn dropped. One can think how monotonous it was to sit all day watching the wheels and jigging this lever. Up high at the back sat the driver, who was not very expert, howling at the mules. They, never very swift, were now intolerably slow; so it took much "dog-gorning" and much "hickorying" to make them get up, and the resulting noise was deafening.

The sun was never so hot and the dust never so unbearable. These were the longest days I ever passed; but at last it was finished and the eighty devoured acres were planted again. George said it was useless work,—everybody's corn was a foot high or more, no corn could ripen after the tenth of June; but we had hopes, and, sure enough, he never had a better or a bigger crop. One day we took a drive across the railroad and there we saw everywhere the effects of the army worm. Luckily it appears only at long intervals.

On the prairie, everyone had so many dogs that it was a marvel how they were fed, or, indeed, how they lived. They ate even the corn from the cob, and stole anything that was not under lock. One day when all the men had gone to a neighbouring town to haul corn, we heard a great barking, and the boys rushed in to tell us that the dogs were after one of the recently bought pigs, the first that we had had. When we arrived on the scene they had tasted blood and it was all up with that pig. His ears were off, and he was bitten in many places. I rushed for the butcher-knife, for we all wanted fresh meat even more than the dogs did; and if the pig must be eaten, C. and I thought it best for us to have the benefit.

So, we set the boys to beat off the dogs, and the eldest helped to hold the pig while we stabbed him, vainly trying to hit a vital spot. At last the animal gave up, and C., in the meantime, having heated water, we dragged him to a board and commenced the dreadful job of getting off the hair. Having only seen it done, we made not the neatest work of it. All the while the fight between the boys and the dogs, occasionally helped with a dash of water, was going on. The combined efforts of all were needed to mount that slippery plank and get the pig under cover from the dogs. When George returned, his indignation at seeing one of his pet pigs lying on that floor was strange to see; but when he learned the truth he sat down beside the departed beast and laughed till we thought he would never end.

One night the doctor was called to a neighbour's where the woman was "very bad," the girl who brought the message said. In the morning, he asked me to go to see her; so, I mounted behind him on the mare, and, though the mud was so deep that I thought it impossible to get there, we at last arrived. The cabin contained only one room; in it were two beds and two trundle-beds; eight children were sitting around a stove burning the hoof off of some pig's-feet, and the room, of course, was filled with their vile odour. The mother lay on the bed, clad in a prairie sunbonnet and a calico wrapper; beside her lay a little, red baby with a piece of fat bacon in its mouth. This was always the manner of treating babies there, she told me. She had a very long hickory stick beside her, and when the children quarrelled she brought it down on them with, "You Mary Ann," or, "You Susan Jane," reducing them to order at once. I asked her to take off her bonnet, but she said that if she did it would give her rheumatism in her head. She never took it off except when eating. Whatever else a prairie woman or child lacks in costume it is never a sunbonnet. When I came to know this woman better I found her to be one of the finest nature. She was a "poor white" from Virginia; but she was so true in all her relations in life, so generous, and always seeking to do a kindness.

At this time the news was most discouraging, the papers full of remorse of war, and so many people about us poor whites from the South, nearly all of them being Rebels, that it was anything but cheerful. The post-office was four miles away; and often many days went by without letters or papers; and now and then such appalling news came that I wonder we could enjoy anything. Soon the rumours of war were confirmed with the news of Fort Sumter and the terrible affair of Bull Run. I immediately wrote to all the people of influence I knew, begging them to procure me some place in the war as nurse, or whatever I could do. Then I waited and waited for a year before I could learn how to get a position; for down there no one seemed to know how to do anything.

Finally, I determined to go back to Massachusetts and find some way to work for the soldiers. That year of waiting is as a blank to me;

we heard nothing but discouraging rumours, and were all so poor. The crops were good enough, but there was no way to get them to market, for the railroad was in the possession of the military. We had two years crop on hand, and most of the cattle died; so we burned corn all that winter. It seemed so wicked. When I started for the East I for the first time realised the war in seeing regiments departing from every city, and in finding it almost impossible to get anywhere.

Arrived in Boston, I appealed immediately to Miss Dix, who promised to place me at once, but who delayed so long that I was beginning to doubt her, when the summons came to start for Washington. This was on Saturday, and Monday night I must leave; so, everybody helped, and I was at the station in time to join my escort. This was in August of 1862.

Chapter 3

Mary Von Olnhausen's recollections of the Civil War are contained in the *Autobiography* before referred to and in letters written to her relatives at home. The first is fragmentary, far from consecutive, and, as would be inevitable, frequently in disagreement with the letters. Those, on the other hand, are seldom dated; and many pages from them, as well as many entire letters, are wanting. Therefore, the narrative is not always unbroken, and the story frequently lacks those salient features which letters written with an eye to publication would have been almost certain to possess. To see the Civil War from the comparatively new point of view of these unstudied sketches is, however, in itself interesting. To read through these artless pictures the strong, unselfish character of a noble woman is doubly worthwhile.

A few pages from the *Autobiography* will serve, by their conciseness, as a sort of preface to the more detailed letters which are then to follow.

(FROM THE *AUTOBIOGRAPHY*.)

Miss Dix, who had been appointed by the President head of the army nurses, took me from Washington to Alexandria to the Mansion House Hospital. She told me on the journey that the surgeon in charge was determined to give her no foothold in any hospital where he reigned, and that I was to take no notice of anything that might occur, and was to make no complaint whatever might happen. She was a stern woman of few words.

There seemed to be much confusion about the Mansion House— which before the war was a famous hotel—and every part of it was crowded. She left me in the office and went in search of Dr. S. The sight of the wounded continuously carried through on stretchers, or led in as they arrived from the boats that lay at the foot of the street on which the hospital stood (this was just after that awful Cedar Mountain battle, August 9), seemed more than I could bear, and I thought Miss Dix would never come. At last she appeared, with Dr. S., who eyed me keenly and, it seemed to me, very savagely, and gave me in charge of an orderly to show me to the surgical ward, as it was called. It consisted of many small rooms, with a broad corridor, every room so full of cots that it was only barely possible to pass between them.

Such a sorrowful sight; the men had just been taken off the battlefield, some of them had been lying three or four days almost without clothing, their wounds never dressed, so dirty and wretched. Someone gave me my charges as to what I was to do; it seemed such a hopeless task to do anything to help them that I wanted to throw myself down and give it up. Miss Dix left me, and soon the doctors came and ordered me to follow them while they examined and dressed the wounds. They seemed to me then, and after wards I found they were, the most brutal men I ever saw. They were both volunteers, and one was a converted Jew who was constantly proclaiming it.

So, I began my work, I might say night and day. The surgeon told me he had no room for me, and a nurse told me he said he would make the house so hot for me I would not stay long. When I told Miss Dix I could not remain without a room to sleep in, she, knowing the plan of driving me out, said, "My child "(I was as nearly as old as herself), "you will stay where I have placed you." In the meantime, McClellan's army was being landed below us from the Peninsula. Night and day the rumbling of heavy cannon, the marching of soldiers, the groaning of the sick and wounded were constantly heard; and yet in all that time I never once looked from the windows, I was so busy with the men.

One of the rooms of the ward was the operating-room, and the passing in and out of those who were to be operated upon, and the coming and going of surgeons added so much to the general confusion. I doubt if at any time during the war there was ever such confusion as at this time. The insufficient help, the unskilful surgeons, and a general want of organisation were very distressing; but I was too busy then and too tired for want of proper sleep to half realise it. Though I slept at the bedsides of the men or in a corner of the rooms, I was afraid to complain lest I be discharged. I was horribly ignorant, of course, and could only try to make the men comfortable; but the staff doctors were very friendly and occasionally helped me, and someone occasionally showed me about bandaging, so by degrees I began to do better. The worst doctor had been discharged, much to my joy, but the other one, despite his drinking habits, stayed on. After the morning visit it was no use calling upon him for anything, and I had to rely on the officer of the day if I needed help. I know now that many a life could have been saved if there had been a competent surgeon in the ward.

At this time, the ward was full of very sick men and sometimes two would be dying at the same time, and both begging me to stay with them, so I got little sleep or rest. Moreover, I had no room of my own. Occasionally a nurse would extend the hospitality of the floor in hers, and I would have a straw bed dragged in on which to get a few hours' sleep. This, with a hurried bath and fresh clothes, was my only rest for weeks. It was no use to complain. The surgeon simply stormed at me and said there was no room; while Miss Dix would say, "You can bear it awhile, my child; I have placed you here and you must stay." I was at that time her only nurse in the Mansion House. Later she succeeded in getting rid of all the others and replacing them with her own.

★★★★★★

From the first letter, written from Washington, it would appear that Miss Dix had intended to take this new nurse to Culpeper (to which General Banks corps fell back after Cedar Mountain). Some change of plan, however, led to her going, instead, to the Mansion House Hospital at Alexandria. There she remained until forced, in July, 1863, by a severe attack of dysentery, to ask for a furlough and to seek recuperation with her sisters in Lexington.

> Washington, August, 1862.
> I have just arrived and do not know when I can write again. Miss Dix has just had a telegram that four hundred men lie at Culpeper with wounds undressed and everything waiting. She goes herself and takes me, so already the work has begun. Miss Dix isn't one bit of a dragon or griffin to me. She received me sweetly and right off asked me to go with her. Help me with your prayers and good wishes. I shall try my best to make you feel I'm not sent in vain.

The following record of the first six or seven weeks of her experience gives but a faint idea of what Mary von Olnhausen encountered in that eventful time. With no experience of serious wounds and with no knowledge of nursing beyond what she had gained in her ministrations to those among her family and friends who had been ill, she was plunged, without preface, into a crowded hospital during one of the bloodiest campaigns of the Civil War. When she arrived at the Mansion House, she had to make her way through a double procession, one of seriously wounded men being taken in, the other of dead being carried out. With no easy and gradual preparation, but on that very night, she was called upon to assist at capital operations performed with little or no anaesthetic, by surgeons who, naturally brutal, had been made doubly so by the hurry of overwork and the magnitude of their seemingly endless task. The operating-room was literally a sea of blood, and its operators had become little better than butchers.

To conditions so adverse were added a hostile atmosphere and a disorganised service, or, rather, a service that had never yet been organised. To those who know or remember only the splendid results of the war and the nobility of self-sacrifice which made these results possible, it is difficult to believe how rankly political corruption, favouritism, and jobbery flourished in the Civil War, above all in the years of its beginning. This hospital especially, in the outskirts of Washington where had gathered all the harpies and vultures of the political camp, was at that time filled with political henchmen and their satellites, more eager for profit than for the binding up of wounds.

Superadded to this corruption was the inevitable disorder and inefficiency inseparable from the organising of a conflict so stupendous by a country unused to war. And this unorganised, this overworked, this more or less corrupt hospital staff was a unit in only one direction,—that of hatred towards women nurses and of determination to "make it so hot" for them as to render it impossible for them to remain. To learn the profession of nursing, to bring order out of chaos, to overcome the unreasonable prejudice of men brutalised by the horrors of a crude and hurried surgery was the task that Mary von Olnhausen had before her; and one can easily accept her apologies for writing this "growling" (as she calls it) letter.

September 21, 1862, Sunday afternoon.

At last I have a few moments that are really my own and a room, too, to sit in that is really mine, and I'm so glad to be alone and writing you. I have been so happy to get your two letters telling me about you all and especially about that box;—you can have no possible idea of the good it will do. I know what all the Sanitary committees in the North have done and how much they think the poor soldiers are comforted; but I can assure you that in the way of delicacies they get mighty little,—none in fact,—and, so far, not even good, nourishing food. As I told the Inspector General a few days since, both in quality and quantity it is intolerable. While they are feeding a thousand outsiders (which was the case during the passing through of the troops and the coming of the wounded), it was excusable; but at no other time. The day before he came bean soup was sent up so salty that no one could swallow a second spoonful; the beef tea was in the same state; and the beans were so hard that all would have had cholera *morbus* if they could have eaten them.

Moreover, the cooks are so overbearing that it is like begging for life to get a thing for the really sick ones who cannot eat common diet. Yet the nurses are obliged to do all extra cooking and are not allowed the use of anything but tin cups or plates; and if we ask for spoon or knife or milk or eggs, you better hear the fuss! The kitchen is a perfect Babel at meal-times, and, rather than encounter the noise, every day I buy eggs and milk, in fact almost every nice thing for the sick ones. I know I have a right to them here; but I've learned enough to know that all who make complaints to headquarters are not only unpopular there but are pitched into by all the house; so, I just speak to nobody, get what I can, and buy the rest.

Sometimes I can *make* eyes at the ice-box man and he'll give me a bit of chicken and mutton; but he isn't always to be melted any more than his ice, though he is the only one who really seems to work for the soldiers. He's quite a character, and is the only man from Dr. S. down who doesn't swear. I'm so disgusted with this last that I think nothing is to be so longed for as to be delivered from swearing,—it's worse than temptation. Now you'll think I am writing a real growling letter; but I know you want to know all, and Mrs. J.'s remarks that we live so fine are utterly groundless. Her husband laughed well at them.

Our bill-of-fare has been unvaried from the time we came till now (I mean at the nurses table); almost always sour bread, and always the worst possible butter, and coffee that can be imagined (I am speaking of breakfast), with sometimes a bit of tough, overdone steak, often no milk, and sometimes no butter. At dinner invariably worse beef, very much done, sometimes potatoes and sometimes not, and once in a while sweet potatoes, which, you know, I hate (but I always claim my share, as

I can take it to some poor fellow in my ward), together with, about once a week, a small piece of pie. Twice we have had a change of baked salt pork instead of beef. For supper, there are always the same sour bread and butter and *such* tea;—and this is all. Today I went out and begged a little mutton soup. The cook gave me some, growling, and said it was only made for the sick. When I tasted it, I thought it was too poor for the well. They say we are going to have a grand reform, that at Washington there is to be a bill-of-fare issued and strictly enforced.

Then what we eat is as nothing to how we eat. We eat with all the cooks and kitchen attendants, and to appreciate them you must once see and hear them. Sometimes I think I cannot bear it another hour, that I'll just leave here; but when I see these miserable nurses and more miserable attendants who are here merely for the poor pay, I think it cruel to go, for, if anywhere, I can do some good here; these poor fellows have at least some-one to help them. All about the house say I'm so proud, and I always intend to be; but in my ward the sick men do not think so, and the blessings and thanks I get from them are all I care for. They, every one, seem as fond of me as if I belonged to them, and I wish you could hear them talk as I sit by their dying beds. Every man except one has died so happy; and he, poor fellow, was so afraid he would die that at last he frightened himself into it. He was a young sergeant from Ohio, only nineteen, and it was so pitiful to see him; but, mercifully, he was unconscious for some hours before his death. His father wrote me such a sorrowful letter.

★★★★★★

(From the *Autobiography*.)

Someone once wrote to me to tell her of the different deathbeds I had witnessed, especially of the deathbed repentances. I can only say that, with the exception of two, none of all my men was afraid to die. I don't remember one who ever expressed repentance; many wished to live, but all seemed to die without fear of the future. The saddest thing about a death in the hospital is the immediate removal of the body. The attendants come with the white sheet which so closely enfolds them, they are silently taken to the dead-house, and the work goes on as if they had never been. Next morning the empty bed, fresh for another patient, is the only reminder of the past night.

★★★★★★

One man sent for me in the middle of the night to come and make his will. He took the ring from his finger for his sister, and his watch and money and notes, and had three other patients witness it. He read it aloud to them in such a clear, loud voice, and pretty soon he died. I read the Bible to him, and he prayed so good; he said he was glad to die, for he never could pray before and his sister wanted him so much to be a Christian.

The poor little boy that I told you had lockjaw died such an awful death. He dictated a pretty boy letter to his mother,—it would have gone right to your heart. He said:

> You told me, mother dear, I'd either come home a cripple or dead; but, mother, I couldn't stay home and see all those noble boys go away to be shot and me staying home and not helping too; but I killed the Rebel who shot me, so he can't kill another boy. He came around the tree after I fell and then I took good aim and killed him.

He was such a dear little country boy, so good and natural; he said: "I'd like to live real well, but then if I can't, I'll try to die and not make any more fuss than I can help;" but, poor fellow, he couldn't help it. He wasn't seventeen. Colonel Hildreth, the man who exposed the swill milk, brought him from the field, (probably that of the second Bull Run), after he had lain there four or five days. He took an ambulance and himself alone drove through all and brought back a load of them.

Did not our government do shamefully to let so many lie there and die? I am so indignant I can't hear of it. It was shameful, and here these surgeons from Boston did all they could to get leave to go to the field, and were denied. It was too awful; you can't realise it unless you were here to see them, as I have, brought in after such suffering. One old Scotchman in my ward lay six days and seven nights, and had only water that the Rebels would now and then give him, and nothing to eat all that time. Yesterday symptoms of lockjaw appeared, and he will soon die of it.

But now comes one of my great troubles;—you know I was placed in a ward that had no female nurse for a long time, and only a horrid, wicked man for a ward master. He treated the patients too cruelly; first thing I did was to have him sent to his regiment,—it's so painful to know there are such bad men for soldiers. The ward was dirtier than you can know, and not one decent attendant, though the largest ward in the house. I've told you how I worked; all the sickest I had charge of. About four weeks ago came a nurse who said she had been in the Crimea,—at any rate she was English and had been fourteen years in hospitals. They gave her a back, upstairs ward. She, of course, knows about bandaging and all that; but, like all old hospital nurses, is no nurse otherwise.

She is the one I had to room with. I almost preferred no bed, as at first; but I would not say one word, it seems so selfish to complain here. Last week, just as I was congratulating myself how well all went and that the wards were so clean and or- derly, up came Dr. S. and thundered out: "Madam, I intend to remove you; I intend Mrs. R. to have this ward; this is the most important one in the house and I consider her the most splen- did nurse in the country; and, by ———, those are the kind of women I intend to fill this house with."

You may judge how bad I felt to leave those men I had had right from the field, and they so fond of me and good; they felt just as bad as I did. It was sweet to hear so many "God bless you's" and assurances that I had saved their lives. I really believe them, for the doctor of the ward was the most negligent, disa- greeable, swearing man I ever met, and left everything to me. Just as I was departing we heard a fearful noise in the entry, and along was dragged my lady, by two officers, dead drunk and swearing like a trooper. So that's the way she took possession of her new ward! I think my exit was better than her entrance. This, of course, made the poor fellows feel ten times worse; and whenever I slip in to see them now there are many tearful eyes, and they beg me so to come back.

You see I did everything for them,—cooked them good things, watched with them nights whenever they needed me, and nev- er left my ward except to eat or sleep; and they (a sister of hers has come to help her, and they are both of a piece) are never there,—just go over the wounds once or twice a day and do nothing more. I acknowledge their superiority in bandaging; but even there I am getting even with them; already the sur- geon-general has praised mine. My new place can't interest me like the old one. I try to do for all alike, but my heart is there most of the time. You may think it strange that I do not leave such a house; but I talked with the chaplain, who is a Massachusetts man and such a Christian, and he begs me to stay here, says I must remember I came for the soldiers, not myself, and here I can do more good than anywhere else.

★★★★★★

(FROM THE AUTOBIOGRAPHY)

I must speak at this time of our Chaplain (Rev. Henry Hopkins, now President of Williams College). Without him I think I could not have gone through the trials I had to bear. Without exception, he was the truest friend and Christian and the bravest man I ever knew. Night and day, he was ready and willing to attend the men, listen to their complaints, write their letters, and comfort them in their last hours. Many a sorrowing one at home must have been comforted by his words written from these death beds. He had a terrible experience at the second Bull Run battle field, where our men lay for many days without food or water, the ground being in the hands of the enemy.

After long pleading, the authorities gave him a pass and ambulance to go through the lines, but he had neither escort nor surgeon. He started at nine o'clock at night with, I think, twenty ambulances. It was raining hard, the roads over which the army had so recently passed were in a frightful state, and he had to go on horseback the distance of fifty miles. It was almost impossible to keep the train together, many of the drivers were drunk, and some would fall asleep, letting their horses stop and blocking those behind. So, he must ride backward and forward the whole night. In the early morning he arrived, and what a sight of sorrow met him!

Of course, all the rebels, both wounded and dead, had been removed; but our men lay as they had fallen, days before. He began his search, and this, he said, was the hardest task of his life, to decide whom to leave and whom to bring away. Of course, he could bring only those able to bear such a journey. The others must be left. Think what a situation for them and himself, every one begging so to be taken! The men worked well in loading the wagons, for they were anxious to get home, having had nothing to eat, since everything the chaplain had with him was distributed among those he must leave behind. After praying with the poor fellows, he started on his weary journey back. All that day he rode backward and forward, hearing only the groans of the wounded and the oaths of the drivers, and did not arrive at the hospital again until nine o'clock at night. I shall never forget his weary face. The poor fellows he brought needed every comfort, and nearly all the night was passed in caring for them.

******

In the next letter reference is made to Lexington as a source of supply for the hospital. This is a good place, therefore, to insert those extracts from the Autobiography which bear upon the work of the devoted women of that town. (An interesting account of the work of these active women is given by Miss Hudson in the *Proceedings of the Lexington Historical Society,* Vol. II. p. 197.) Their ceaseless labours and unstinted generosity enabled Mrs. von Olnhausen to do much for her soldiers that otherwise would have been impossible; and she never failed to give those ladies full credit for their share in her work. Indeed, so generous was her nature, that she perhaps assigned to them a larger measure of credit than they would have cared to claim. She, to whom most of the product of their busy hands went, says of them:—

(FROM THE *AUTOBIOGRAPHY*)

I had constantly been receiving comforts of all kinds for the sick and wounded in my care from my kind friends at home. These I had always kept in my own room (now I had one), giving them, when needed, to the sick in other wards as well as to those in my own. One day the head surgeon sent for me, and said he heard I was in the habit of receiving such things, and that he had determined in future to have all such boxes sent to the dispensary and distributed from there. Therefore, all such things as I had in my possession must be sent there at once. I told him all I had came from my personal friends in Lexington, and sooner than have them given to his drunken dispensary clerks to be eaten and drank and used by them, I would throw them out upon the pavement.

He said the complaint was constantly made that my men were better served and cared for, and petitions were constantly made to be admitted there on that account. I assured him that I always divided with all who really needed them. Then he told me there was an order addressed to me for a number of barrels of apples lying at the wharf, that they were needed for the hospital, and that I must give an order for them to be sent to him at once. "No," I said, "those are for myself, and I shall send them back unless I can do with them what I choose." So, I bade him *adieu* and flew back to my room, expecting every moment some new development.

Soon came another summons to the office. He asked if I had changed my mind, as an order had come that the apples must be at once sent for. I told him "No."

"Well, what will you do with them?"

"Have them sent to my ward and from there distributed, unless you will give me a store room where they can be safely locked and the key put in my charge."

After a moment he asked, if he would do that, would I be willing to place my own stores there and take charge and distribute them as they were needed. I answered, "No, I was there to dress wounds and care for the soldiers personally, and I was too busy to do it and take charge of my ward." He became angry and asked me to suggest someone to whom I would be willing to give the room. A few days before Miss Dix had brought to the hospital a widow whom I could trust, so I suggested her; and after much talk the thing was settled. Meantime he gave me a room for the apples; so, by night they were stored. Then I sent to every ward a barrel, one to the cooks and one to the doctor. They were a splendid lot, and so welcome, for we had had only very little fruit and every one craved it. Very soon the store-room was a fixed fact, and I had the comfort of knowing that the whole house enjoyed what was meant for the soldiers.

Lexington came to be a very dear place to all I cared for. I am sure many who read these papers will remember the name with gratitude even without its sacred associations. It was such a delight to receive a box from Lexington, and the expectation of what had come was so great that I usually made a little feast for the men's tea. I always identified myself with Lexington, and never can enough thank that little band of good women who gave me the opportunity to do so much good. Their interest never flagged. Till the very end of the war every month brought com forts from them. A soldier never went from my ward, either to his regiment or to his home, without some proper clothing and often a little money to help him on the journey. For this I take no credit; it was only through those dear friends I was able to do it.

Wednesday (October, 1862),

Tonight, for supper, I have made some butter cakes for my men, and such a glorious hash; and won't they think I'm the best woman in the house? They do, anyway; you ought to hear them brag! I know old Lexington would be real glad. I made gruel in my little saucepan the first thing this morning. The cook flew at me as I was going out of the kitchen: "Here, you can't take that upstairs; it's against the rules." I wanted to say "darn the rules," but I only said, "It's mine, I thank you," and I felt big. I am always running against some of their rules; but it's hard keeping the run, they have so many. Now I don't "say it for say," but no bandages are like yours. I can do an arm or leg forty times as well with them, and we are likely to want all we have if the report is true of the big battle. I dread to see the house filled again with more poor sufferers. You would be amused to hear me entertaining them in the evening. I go the whole rounds, taking my little camp-stool, or kneeling beside their beds. They all treat me with such confidence. I know all their histories and sorrows; they talk just like I was their mother. How I do wish I were real good and pious; I could do so much then.

The remaining extracts from her letters for the year 1862 are fully characteristic of this impulsive, warm-hearted, enthusiastic, not always dis criminating woman. Her denunciations of the Post Camp (of which the "fever camps" of the Spanish-American War seem to have been a mild repetition), her personal affection for all her patients, her unhesitating hospitality, the results of which make her "bawl," her good-natured ridicule of her guests and of herself picture Mary von Olnhausen just as she was and as she remained to the end of her long life. She wore her heart and her frank, open character upon her sleeve, and many were the unworthy daws who profited thereby.

Alexandria, November 9, 1862.
Did I tell you that Governor Andrew was here one day, and in my ward, too? I was so sorry to miss him; but, as usual, when anybody comes I'm cooking. He talked "bunkum" to the Massachusetts boys; they all felt so proud, and it made the other boys quite jealous.
I wish you could look into my ward tonight and see these miserable sick men who have come in from the convalescent camp during the last week. Such wrecks I never saw, all worn out with fever and diarrhoea or some other chronic complaint; it's worse than wounded men. This horrid camp is about a mile from here and is such a place! Several thousand have been there, just lying on the ground in tents, many without blankets, none

with more than one, the worst possible food to eat, and growing sicker and dying every day. Your heart would ache forever after if you could once see them. All discharged from the hospitals, both here and at Washington, are sent out there; it's called the Post Camp. Men just getting up from wounds, fevers, and other sickness, men who have been confined for months in hospitals without any exercise or exposure, when pronounced fit to join their regiments, are sent out there to await orders. Some of them lie for weeks there, not being able to learn where their regiment is or even to get transportation to it. These are sure to get sick again, and many of them die. The camp is so disorganised that it's almost impossible to find a man after he once gets into it.

One night last week, about nine o'clock, five of these men were sent to me, and I had but three empty beds. Five such objects I never saw,—three with typhoid, one German with shaking palsy, and one with paralysis. They told me they had been pronounced fit for duty and sent out there, where they had been for three weeks or more, every day growing sicker. The night before it had rained steadily and they just lay in pools of mud. What can our government be doing to let such a place exist? Two of them have already died and one of the others, I fear, will. The Massachusetts man (from Plymouth) was brought up in a smaller man's arms, like a baby; so you can think how thin he was. He had his senses, and talked so much about getting home and his "Carry," it was just too pitiful. The chaplain wrote to her for him, and again after his death.

He and a young man from New York both died last Sunday night; the other one never had his senses after he came in, so we could find nothing out about him; but he was always talking of his mother; and when I called him Charlie he said, "That's what mother called me; she always said Charlie." He seemed to want me with him all the time, would look around for me and get right out of bed to follow me as soon as I left him. They lay at extreme ends of the ward, so I just ran from one to the other all day. One died at eight and the other at nine o'clock, so I could be with both. I never leave a man to sleep or to eat when I think he will soon die; it seems at least as if a woman ought to close these poor fellows' eyes; no mother or wife or sister about them. I feel that I must be all to them then, and the last words of many dying men have been thanks for what I have done. It is so splendid to be able to do anything for them; I do not lose my interest or enthusiasm one bit. Everybody said, when I first came, "Oh, you'll get over this after a while and be hard just like us," but I never can. If possible, I feel more than then.

Such a pleasant thing happened today. It was snowing, and I was on my knees trying to make my fire burn, when came a knock, and in walked a young man. I thought I'd seen his face, but still it was so changed, I could not place him; he had to tell me who he was. He was one of the Culpeper boys who left for some Northern hospital the first of September. He was wounded through the body, and was very sick while under my care. He had just got back to the Post Camp to join his regiment, and came at once to see and thank me. The tears ran down his cheeks when he told me how he missed my care and how sick he had been since he left here.

His wound reopened and fever ensued, and for three days he did nothing but call for Miss Mary (that's what they call me, my name is so hard). When he came to his senses they all bothered him so; but he told them he could never be shamed for that; I was the best nurse and the best woman he knew, and if all the nurses were like me many a poor boy would get well who had died. He says that all the other boys who went at that time said the same. Of course, I felt real grateful, but I think the feeling was more for my friends and Lexington than for myself. I should so hate to disappoint them, and am so proud when I make them a pleasure.

One morning last week I heard that the First Massachusetts and all that division were moving; so, I asked Dr. Stewart for an ambulance and went out to the camp, hardly hoping that I should see them, as all said I would be too late. How glad I was I went! It was the finest sight I ever saw. Far and near they were breaking camp, and from a high hill we saw the whole division in motion; it was grand. We had a chance to speak to everybody we knew, and to bid them goodbye. They expected a fight immediately, but as yet we have not heard of them. It made me sad enough, though, to see them all going. I thought how many of them would never come back. They were in splendid spirits longed for a fight the best kind. That's the only time I've been out of the house since I wrote you last.

The disastrous Battle of Fredericksburg, with its great number of killed and wounded, took place on December 13. Worn out with excitement and fatigue, and justly indignant at the inadequacy of the preparations for caring for the suffering men, Mrs. von Olnhausen wrote:

Monday night (December 15, 1862). Today has been such an awful day, bringing in the wounded from Frederick. The whole street was full of ambulances, and the sick lay outside on the sidewalks from nine in the morning till five in the evening. Of course, places were found for some; but already the house was full; so, the most had to be packed back again and taken off to Fairfax Seminary, two miles out. I have been so indignant all day,—not a thing done for them, not a wound dressed. To be sure, they got dinner; but no supper. They reached town last evening, lay in the cars all night without blankets or food, were chucked into ambulances, lay about here all day, and tonight were put back into ambulances and carted off again. I think every man who comes a-soldiering is a fool!

Sunday night (December, 1862). This has been as blue a week as ever I passed. Tuesday night (I mean Tuesday week) two women arrived, one to see her sick son and the other her husband; one came from western Wisconsin and the other from northern New York. Dr. S. had just made a new law forbidding visitors to stay in the house; but they were so very poor, and had come so far and felt so bad, I could not bear to see them. So, I, bold as a sheep, really decided to face the doctor and to beg him to let them stay. At first, he said decidedly, "No;" but you know how I hang on and grow braver; so finally,—to get rid of me, I guess—he said, "Yes, if you will take them into your own room."

Oh, dear! now I had just got so nicely settled and so snug; but of course, I could not refuse, and would not, under the circumstances. One of them is very sweet, but the other is a real prairie woman, all but the sunbonnet. Thursday night came a new woman, from western Massachusetts. Dr. S. sent for me and asked if I had any objection to receiving this Mrs. M. as sharer of my room, since there was no unoccupied room fit for her at present. He seemed to forget that I had two ladies already hidden there. Of course, I had to take her, although I did hate it so bad. So that night we had four, and only bedding for two, and the room not large. Next morning the Wisconsin man died, and his wife left that night; but before she left down came Miss Dix with two nurses, one to superintend the low diet and one as nurse; as doctor was not in, and she must return to Washington, she begged me to take charge of them till his return.

Now here were six of us, and my gentleman not returned when night came! I managed to find two empty beds in the ward to put them in, but all day Sunday imagine my utter despair! All of them sitting here the whole day, and Monday and Tuesday; who could write? I only felt like bawling. I could not keep the room decent, and they all looked so forlorn and, mind you, they had to furnish their own food and cook it themselves, so my stewer was always going. I could not wash or dress, or in fact do anything; and the ward is kept so cold I could not sit anywhere with comfort. I had so many errands to do for them I was quite worn out.

At last, Wednesday, Dr. S. came; one nurse he rejected, the other he retained; and to Mrs. M. he assigned a ward; but we were still four,—all widows, all old, and all but me exceedingly pious, and ministers widows at that. Sometimes we would have jolly laughs, though, for all the trouble; and Mrs. B., the one who will take charge of the cooking, is lovely, just such a woman as I like. Yesterday, Mrs. B. got her room, and out of pity to me she let Mrs. M. sleep in it. So, I expected to have at least a bed again; when, just at dark, came in another nurse with a note from Miss Dix to please give her Sunday quarters. So, I took the blanket again and don't mean to expect any more peace; they have everyone been sitting here all day, and I had to wait for them to go to bed to get a chance at you.

We have been sending off this week everyone who could be moved; and you may believe it's been a pretty blue time with me, I have had so many of them so long under my care. All have been sent to New York on the *Daniel Webster*; thanks to that last splendid box, I have been able to make many of them comfortable. Not one left without some warm garments. I expect they will suffer much as it is, but I'm glad they are getting near home. Poor fellows! some of them are so lean and miserable.

Chapter 4

Arriving at the Mansion House Hospital in August of 1862, Mrs. von Olnhausen seems to have conquered the prejudices of the surgical staff by the beginning of 1863. Therefore, that year was to prove a happier one. The long strain of work, however, together with the evil climate of Washington, brought upon her, in June, 1863, a serious attack of dysentery. This so reduced her that she was obliged to ask for a furlough and to return, with some of her relatives who had come for her, to Lexington.

Her letters during this first half of 1863 need little comment. They chronicle, in her amusing way, the conciliation of her first head-surgeon and the coming of a successor; her temporarily successful but eventually disastrous warfare with a most "unjust steward;" and the varying duties and pleasures of her busy life.

> Alexandria, Sunday evening (January, 1863).
>
> I suppose you just think I never am going to write again; but I can't help it, I live in such a state of confusion all the time. There is always somebody new quartered upon me. I have had a "game" leg and so many bad sick ones, and now I have lost one poor boy. His death was such a mystery to me, for when he did not die of lockjaw, which I expected from the appearance of the wound, I could not believe how he could die so soon.
>
> ★★★★★★

The use of "when" for "if," which is found so often in her letters, was caught evidently from Mr. von Olnhausen, who could not rid himself of the German *wenn*. Other German words and idioms crop out frequently in her letters, especially in those written during her residence in Saxony.

> ★★★★★★

He died Saturday; and the Tuesday after, at noon, came his poor father and mother. It was dreadful to have to tell them he was dead and buried. I never witnessed more intense grief; for he was their only boy, and they were so proud of him. But he was the wickedest boy I have ever seen die; almost his last breath was an oath; and I could not make him say one word for his father or mother. I tried so hard to make him talk of them. How his poor mother did long to have one word from him; I had to invent a bit just to make her a little comfort. They were such nice, respectable people; and stayed until Friday,—in my room all the time. You may think how they were in my way, though I could not say "No" to them.

You will be glad to know the change in Dr. S.'s treatment of me. I guess he finds it is creditable to him to have some ladies around. He is most polite when he meets me; and the night we were expecting the wounded he came to my door and asked me to go through my ward with him. It was nine o'clock, but the rooms did look nice, the beds all so clean, and clothes for each man laid out, such bright fires and warm and cold water, sponges and everything else ready. He was so pleased, and said he had found no other ward in such order. Then he turned and asked me if he might come to my room for a few moments, he had something to say to me.

When there he told me, he had reason to believe that I thought he did not like me, and he himself knew he had been sometimes rude to me, for which he apologized. "But, madam, you are mistaken; I am more than satisfied; I would have you leave on no account; you have done and are doing more to elevate the tone of this hospital than any one in it, and anything you ask for your ward or for yourself I will grant; only always come to me; don't send through a third person." Now this was real nice, wasn't it? Everybody likes to be appreciated. He said, too, he had been watching me for a long time and knew all I'd done,—"and more than that, every doctor and every man in the house likes you."

I wish you could hear his voice; it is about three times louder than a bull's. He said he knew people called him a Rebel; but he denied the charge stoutly and spoke right feelingly of his honour to the flag. He finally declared, "With you and Mrs. B., madam, this house shall be the first hospital in the country;" and you have no idea what a change there is here since she came. She is matron, has the sole charge of the low diet—which is the most important in the house—so we are entirely relieved of that horrid cooking; and she does make such nice things, all sorts of delicious delicacies, that one can see the men improve. She is a most interesting woman and has had such a sad life. Her only boy was killed in the army. She was at Antietam when her son-in-law came to tell her that her boy was dead. From that moment, she was stark mad; they took her home to Chambersburg, forty miles; she was so bad that the next day they took her, by all the doctors' advice, to the asylum at Harrisburg, her daughter and son-in-law going with her. While they were making arrangements for her entrance, she was temporarily placed in the room where all the worst insane were, and there she came to her senses,—just think of it, her full and entire senses! She turned to the doctor and said, "Doctor, they have brought me to a mad-house; what is this for?"

He tried to soothe her; she demanded to see her daughter; but they supposed it was another phase, so the daughter went off without seeing her at all, fearing to injure her. She was taken to her room, and there were two women always with her night and day, everybody supposing her insane and paying no heed to her. She demanded to go home; of course, they would not let her, and there she was kept ten days with her terrible grief for her dear boy and in this awful life.

Then she told her daughter, in a letter, that when she did not come immediately and take her home she would disinherit her and never see her again while she lived. Of course, the poor girl came and took her right away, though the doctor opposed her; but she saw at once that her mother was entirely sane. Mrs. B. stayed in Chambersburg two days and then came right to Miss Dix, who treated her so tenderly and beautifully, keeping her busy now in one hospital, now in another, till she was over the worst of her grief and her health was established. Then she brought her here for good.

We had quite an entertainment New Year's night (quite stupid, I mean). Of course, all the doctors made lengthy speeches, and then there was tremendous howling of patriotic songs. There were lots of outside ladies, all dressed up fine, in front; and, for the patients, a cake big as a cart wheel and heavy as lead, which was capital. G. will remember how fond I am of cake with a "stripe," though I don't think it is the best diet for sick people.

Alexandria (January or February, 1863).
I'm sure you will be surprised at my long letter to the Society
(Lexington Soldiers Aid Society), and, after all, so little that is
satisfactory said in it; but you know just how hard it is for me to
write duty letters. Do look over the spelling, especially Pyemia.
I don't know if it should have a *y* or an *i* in it. I only spelled
it as it sounds. You see one word was wrong in the very first;
there may be a dozen. When you think I have said too much
you might condense it; I could, now it is done, only I have no
time to copy.

Do give me some clue to the P. family. I have a vision of old P.;
what is he? I can't place him, but somehow it seems like he was
connected with L. in some funny way. Did she ever have him
for a pet *chore man* (I wrote it "chaw" first)? Anyway, the poor
boy looks bad enough. I don't exactly fancy the hospital he is
in; but his bed looked clean and I guess he is well taken care of.
I promised to go and see him every day, so I shall. How I wish
he could have been with me! I would have felt so proud to have
a Lexington soldier in my care.

Do you know, I grow just as mean as a pig with my things! I
won't give a single well man a thing, only those who are going
off to camp. It's come to be a regular thing for all the clerks
and detailed men about the house to ask for this or that; but
I always tell them, "No, they are sent for the sick soldiers and
not for well men shirking duty and lying around hospitals!" I
used not to be so savage, but I have got perfectly disgusted with
these men. They are just too lazy to do duty, and so get big pay
and "laze" around. There are so many invalids who could do all
they do, and they might be fighting. When you could once see
the abuse! Look into the kitchen, for instance, and see the great,
strong men who are cooking; then you'd be mad, too!

Isn't it too bad the apples have not come? I feel so disappointed,
but Dr. S. is sharp after them. He, by the way, is good as pie
to me. Speaking of pies, you did not send me one; but *them*
dough nuts and that *there* square gingerbread was too *dolicious*.
I feel pretty mean about giving the last, and the first we ate in
our own room. My brains are baked in my head, but I've got
wound up and it's one dem'd grind now. The fire is so hot, and
if I move my chair one inch the leg will come out. It's a "com-
pound comminuted fracture" and takes too much time to set

43

it often.

Alexandria, February, 1863.
I must tell you about a little excursion we made on the 14th.
Dr. S. gave us leave (Mrs. B. and me) to go down to Mt. Vernon
with some of our men. He said we could take but twelve,—as
the tug could get only within a mile of the shore,—and that
we must row in a small boat. First, we must take those who had
been longest wounded and after that all the amputations. He
gave us a little tug to go in, the best and fastest on the river, and
I wish you could have seen us set off, seven pairs of crutches. It
would have done your heart good to see how happy the poor
fellows were; think! for six months some of them had been
shut up and had hardly stepped on the ground. They were just
as gay with us old nurses as if we had all been young. I told
them, coming home, that the only omission, for St. Valentine's,
had been that nobody had asked us to marry him; so, they all
began at once. The one-legs had the best of it, for they are sure
of eight dollars a month.
I thought I might be able to tell you a little of Mt. Vernon and
my impressions, but that would be impossible. I'm convinced
that one ought to be alone there, or at least with one's best
friend, everything seems so sacred. You feel that you stand in the
presence of the spirit, at least, of Washington; and I could almost
believe I saw him. It seemed wicked to speak aloud. The rooms
are unfurnished and most desolate, and the old harpsichord
sounds unearthly. The mantel-piece and hearth in the dining
room are splendid. The carving is in strong *bas-relief* to represent
agriculture in all its forms. Would you believe that some vandals
have broken horns from cows, arms from milkmaids, and legs
from dogs and boys to take away as relics? Isn't it shameful? The
view from the front of the house is splendid; such a beautiful
river, with the fort and hills opposite.

Alexandria (March, 1863).
We have been having a general turn-up and turn-out, and so
have much to talk about; every day brings some new thing to
light. Dr. S. is promoted and leaves here for some other field. He
made his farewell tonight and was much affected at parting. He
has been to me as kind as a brother, and has regretted so many
times that he did not know me at first.

Our new doctor in charge is Dr. Page. I don't know where he comes from. I saw him this morning for the first time; he is nice looking and gentlemanly, and I'm particularly pleased, for he found much fault in every ward but mine, and in mine he praised everything. The fact is I have the best attendants in the house, and they will do anything for me; so it is not much praise to me, after all; and then, at present, I have the only sick in the house (I mean badly wounded—and you'd better believe they are well bandaged up inspection days; they *have* to like it). I am quite impatient to know where I shall be located. There was talk of New Mexico and New Orleans; but nobody knows yet. The river is black with ducks; but they are too dear to buy, and I have no time to go shooting. Sometimes in the early morning I can hear all the birds sing; but, after that, these army wagons constantly moving deaden any sound, and not a breath of the country reaches us. Now the lizards and beetles are waking up and I long to be out in it. If the weather would only be warm and pleasant we might go out, now that we have leisure, only the mud is so frightful.

We have just heard that by the last of the week every bed in the house will be full; the sick and wounded are all to be sent from the front. I am sorry the sick are coming; I never want another sick man in my ward; I like all wounded. Don't you feel hopeful now about the war? These reforms are splendid and so needed. I believe now all will go well. How poor the Rebs must be!

I thought it best not to trouble you with an account of how we have been living lately,—everything cut off, nothing but coffee (so poor and with hardly ever milk) and dry bread for breakfast; for dinner bread and meat (and such meat! always the tail or neck or some other nasty part), and at night coffee and bread again. Being hungry is nothing to being so insulted. We knew we had a right to all our rations; and while Dr. S. was here we always urged Mrs. B. to ask him, and so put us out of the power of these cooks. They hate us because we are decent women and will fight for the soldiers' rights, thus cutting off their resources. For some reason, she never would; she thought he would believe us selfish or something.

One day it was past all bearing. I was positively so hungry I could have eaten cat's meat. I sat over the fire after supper, tired and hungry and wondering if the good I did was balanced by my suffering (more from insults than anything else), when all at once it struck me to go to Dr. Page myself. It was eight o'clock; I found him alone, and he listened to all my story. He seemed so surprised at it, said we had not even one privilege we were entitled to, called the steward—who is just the meanest, hatefullest (oh, help me to a word, I don't care if it *is* profane) man that ever lived—and told him that in future we were to draw our own rations and have our own cook. I felt so elated, and when I announced it next morning the women actually embraced me. Well, we waited for five days; no rations, though we kept demanding them. Then we were cut down short enough; deprived even of sugar. Thereupon I sent word to H. (the steward) that when the rations did not come at once I would appeal to Dr. Page again. So, the rations for ten days (that's the time for drawing) came; but there was such a little allowance that we had to buy half we ate. I got some soldiers who had been in the quartermaster's department to look at them; and they said we had not a third of what we ought. So up to Dr. Page I went again and told him of the matter. He called H., who swore we had full weight of everything.

I said, "Doctor, just make us independent of this man; let us draw direct from the Quartermaster."

"Certainly, when you like it;" and he signed our requisition for eight women.

Mrs. B. and I went down, taking a boy along, to bring the rations up. Judge of our consternation when it took a cart to carry them! Eighty pounds of meat, eighty pounds of flour, and so much beans, rice, molasses, vinegar, pork, tea, coffee and sugar,—enough for every luxury. We acted like fools. I was really ashamed to find myself so rejoiced,—even candles. We called all the women down to see, and the cooks were all so mad, knowing we were out of their clutches, they could have bitten us. We went out and traded off sixty-two pounds of meat and got $5.25 for it in cash; this buys our butter and milk. Then our flour we exchange with a baker, pound for pound, so we can have cake and pies sometimes; and we shall keep our beans and rice till we get a bushel of them, and then change them off. Isn't it nice? And yesterday all gave a little, and the rest we took from the five dollars, making enough to get us cups and saucers, white plates and dishes. You can't think how nice our table looked; the luxury of a cup after drinking eight months out of a tin or earthen mug was too much. I would not have anybody I love connected with the Quartermaster and Hospital department for the world; they cannot have power, it seems to me, and be honest; it is proven every day. A good boy comes in and, if he has some talent, is given something to do in that department. From that moment he begins to fall, puts on such airs, and pockets all he can.

When our own battles were settled, then it was time, when good feeding had given us a little strength, to put in for our patients; so last Sunday morning I opened fire. Dr. C. has that department, so I attacked him; but he was mad when I told him the patients would starve only for the nurses, who had to buy everything the sickest men ate. He denied it, and said he knew his nurse did not do it. So, she was called, and said she did; then the others were called; and, at last, we had about every nurse and doctor in the house growling and snarling. Dr. C. said they had everything according to the new diet-table; some of the doctors denied it and some of them backed him up; at last we all adjourned to some underground room (the bread-room) to read the table list, when it proved that they got nothing in the quantity even that was ordered there; and as to quality, Lord help them!

How I wish you could have heard the row! It went on all day; even in the evening everybody was called up and talked to; and the result is that it has been a little better this week, though far from the mark, and soon (if it grows less every day) it will be back to the old standard, for that wretch H. or somebody will miss the money and get it back if possible. So, you see our path is not all rose-leaves, and you can see, too, one of the many impositions put upon the noble fellows who are throwing away their lives for such men as these. Are all men naturally bad? That's going to be the only religious question I shall study in the future. I guess this war will make me religious, for one. I am getting a good deal more patient and for giving than I used to be, but I'll never forgive the soldiers enemies. I can sooner forgive the Rebels who kill them.

You wonder the boys don't answer the notes (written by Lexington ladies and sent with the clothing); you don't know how modest they feel. Then, too, I suppose many of them are not much used to writing. Moreover, they had some rebuffs from that Miss ——; she wrote to them and they answered; and then she thought she would be motherly, advise them about their spelling, etc., and that mortified them. Of course, the letters were shown all around, so it's given them all a holy horror of writing to strange women.

Blue Eyes, my pet boy, leaves me tomorrow; he is too lovely, so confiding and sweet; he is to be discharged. I suppose he cannot walk for a long time, though his wound is quite healed. I shall be bluer than ever when he goes. T., too, goes home tomorrow. I never have told you about him; he is too mean to live. He is dreadfully mad they gave him his discharge; says he meant to stay round the hospital this summer, as it's the easiest way to get $13 a month. He's the first mean Massachusetts man I've met.

Alexandria, Friday (March or April, 1863). I hardly know whether I have a head on my shoulders; since last summer I never saw such times here,—sick coming and going all the time. I've forgotten where I left off and can't think what to tell first. I believe I told you about the amputations we had; those boys were so sick for so long; but that was a hard time! Dr. B. away, and so much resting on me, and such wounds to dress. The arm boy wiggled through and is still alive. He is just as disagreeable as ever; but it is only since four days that we have thought he could live. But that other splendid man dies. I never felt sorrier; he was such a noble fellow and so good and patient. He wanted me by him all the time, and would not let any one touch him but me; he died the Sunday after I wrote last.

The very night he died they "piked" the wounded in upon us from that cavalry fight. They were all badly shot, and the amputations had all been performed on the field. I had an Eighth Illinois boy with the leg off nearly to the body; he was almost pulseless when he came, and was so much exhausted with the long ride that it was twenty-four hours before we could get him warm at all, and he has been lying in a hopeless state ever since. He dictated such a beautiful letter to his sister, though it was almost impossible to keep him awake for more than a minute at a time. He died yesterday morning, and I felt as if half the ward was gone. I had to write his sister; it is so hard to write such letters. He was a better kind of a boy than I was used to seeing in Illinois.

You would have to be here to realise how busy I have been. We have no low-diet cook now since Mrs. B. gave it up, and it's so hard going up and down four long flights of stairs for everything; for we can't even warm a drop of water up here. Often, I make the journey ten or fifteen times a day. If it were not for this, I would like my ward better than any other in the house; but it takes the wind.

You can form no idea of our disturbed nights,—constant alarms and the backward movement of the army. The continual rattling of heavy wagons and the guard patrolling and challenging, one cannot sleep much. I have not felt fully awake in a fortnight; and when the noise outside is a little less, comes the watchman with, "Somebody has a chill, or a pain, or wants to see me," so all nights are disturbed ones. You know what a dumb sort of feeling one has after a succession of such nights; so, you can expect only stupidity from me. Sunday evening was the crowner of all; I never can forget it. We were all day expecting the wounded, all who have been lying down front; those poor, neglected soldiers, some seventeen hundred in all, were brought to this place. Such a dreary sight; the streets perfectly jammed with the poor blessed cripples, ambulances, stretchers, beds, crutches, everything. It was just horrible.

It was twelve o'clock when the last boat-load arrived; the attendants were all tired out with lugging them, and yet there were still hundreds not cared for. Two boat-loads had to be reloaded and sent to Washington. Think of those poor sufferers! I had not a single attendant to do a thing. W. and "Jack the Giant Killer" had them all to wash; and I helped do that and dressed all the wounds besides. I had fractures to put up and anterior splints to make, all without one word of advice. Dr. F. has been my doctor since Dr. B. went; but he has another big ward and was also officer of the day, so could not leave for a moment. He sent for me and said he should leave everything for me to manage as I thought proper. Dr. Page came up about twelve and was so pleased with what I had done. It was nearly morning when we got to bed.

Monday and Tuesday went off splendidly. I had all the work I wanted and such "bully" wounds to dress; but Tuesday night came another despatch from headquarters that every man who could be moved must leave next morning for Philadelphia; so, before I had got interested or could distinguish one man from another I lost them all. They were such a nice set of men, all from the Twelfth and Sixth army corps, and such brave boys; wasn't it too bad when we had got them all cleaned up and straightened out to have them go again? They left me only six of the new cases. I have eleven in all. It was harder to have them go than come, I think; they did not want to leave, either. This has been the most confusing time I have known since last summer. Mrs. B. is quite worn out; she had so many bad thigh fractures which could not be brought upstairs.

Sunday night (March or April, 1863). I shall give up, I cannot write; I have tried fifty times since this was commenced. You can't know all I have done these last two days; more patients have come and gone, and now I have only ten left in my ward; but I have been into two other wards helping, or rather putting up anterior splints; for you will feel quite proud to know that I can put them up—so the surgeons say—better than anyone in the house. At any rate, Dr. P. of Boston is lying here with his leg very badly fractured; he is not in my ward, but Dr. F. sent compliments for me to come and dress it. He and two other surgeons stood by while I worked; they never gave one word of advice, just stood and looked on; and when I had finished they all said they never saw one so well put up. I felt so glad, for you must see it was no small compliment. The patient himself is a fine surgeon, and he was most delighted of all. I know this sounds very egotistical, but at present my passion is wound dressing, and I *will* excel.

Major Higginson, of the First Massachusetts Cavalry, is in the house. He is such a pleasant man, cousin to the minister; he so wants to come into my ward. His father is here to take him home when he is well enough. Besides three sabre cuts, he has a bullet in him. He asked me to come down every day and see him, for he has such a hateful nurse. He used to be Lieutenant in the Second Massachusetts, Company E. Isn't it provoking I never can get Massachusetts boys in my ward?

I'm in for the war until discharged; I can't for a moment regret it; I could never be contented now at home remembering what I can do here and how many need me. I know that all are not fitted for this life, but I feel as if it were my special calling and I shall not leave it, if God gives me strength, while I know there is a Union soldier to nurse. You can have no idea how one's patriotism grows while one sees those poor fellows lying so piteously. I can't see how such a thing as a Copperhead can live. Do kill everyone in Lexington. How I do wish every one of them was in the Rebel lines to be shot down!

The town is full of rumours today. They say we are having the best of it; but what can one believe? We heard cannonading last night, but far off. I suppose the Second (Massachusetts) is fighting again; it always fights, you know. I don't have any time to enjoy my new clothes; I can't even glance in the glass to see how I look in them. I had my old bonnet "newed" up, and it looks delicious.

Alexandria (April or May, 1863), Wednesday. We went to Washington yesterday, sightseeing,—Mrs. B. and daughter, Mrs. M. and I. We did the Smithsonian thoroughly, and then went to the Capitol; whereupon it commenced raining like piker. We had a fine chance to see everything, for we could not get away, took a lunch there (about the poorest ever was eaten), but had finally to come back again. We have to go again one day this week to finish up the business.

I wish you could see some of the green specimens we met yesterday; it was better than all else. Such shocking, "muggins" women; they had to sit in every chair and stand in every place, and they talked about the piles of babies (cupids and angels) painted on the walls; "didn't see what they painted them there for." They went into all the private rooms and asked so many questions; they "hadn't no umbrel and no gums, and didn't see what they was going to do." I concluded the unterrified democracy had got around, sure. I suppose I seemed just as verdant, but I didn't feel so.

Alexandria, Wednesday (May, 1863). W. has just come back to me wounded in the head. We hope not badly; but he is in a very exhausted state, as when he went into the field he was not fit for it, and they had never stopped marching from Monday morning at three o'clock till Sunday, when he was wounded; just marching and fighting all the time. Poor fellow, he was so overcome when he got here; he is sleeping now, and when he wakes the doctor will examine him, and I shall know better how he is. The glorious Second (Massachusetts) has won new laurels. He says he would rather have been the meanest private in that than a general anywhere else. This is a bad storm for our poor fellows, but let us hope for the best. I feel sure we shall win. How I hate my Reb wounded; they are so exultant, too, this morning; I'm sure they have heard something. I don't think I can dress their wounds any more. Aunt Mary S. asked them if they were well treated. "Oh, splendid, madam."

"I am glad to hear it," she said, "I like even my enemies to be well treated."

"Oh, madam, you are not Secesh then?"

"No, sir, not a drop of traitor blood runs in my veins." She looked bully when she said it.

There is a lot of fun made about turning the boxes over to the hospital. Today one of the nurses was telling her doctor of my box and the fine dresses it contained; she is rather "soft," and said I had such a lovely lawn and a Balmoral skirt she wanted. So, he wrote an order, and sent it in, for "One purple lawn dress and one Balmoral skirt to be delivered to the nurse on the third floor." It took some time for Mrs. B. to get the matter through her wool.

I'm reading *Les Miserables* to W. to try to make him contented. I read it as I would like to have it read to me, on the jump and skip plan.

A lot of women came in today just as I was dressing "Blue Beard's" wound. One of them, as she saw it, just gave a stagger and fell up against the wall. She was pale as could be, and I thought would faint. All the women crowded around, and one young one said, "Oh, I always thought I should so like to be a nurse." She looked about as much account as a yellow cat.

His wound, by the way, isn't doing very well; but he's such a nice fellow, the *beau ideal* of a soldier in bearing, and looks so prompt and trig, and is real good and patriotic. He wants to go back to the field, but I'm afraid the poor fellow never will. He won't be idle, so he has taken the diet and dispensary books and the light work of the ward. My big Jack is getting better and will soon be off again; he, too, is a real nice fellow. I want to make him wound-dresser, if we ever have any wounded, but he would rather be in the field. Oh, the shirks there are in this army; so many cowards to one brave man!

Alexandria, VA., Sunday, May 17, 1863.
We have been expecting some wounded all day from Fairfax Station; there was a fight with the Guerillas and Vermont cavalry and some New York regiment; but they have not come yet; probably, as usual, they will come in the night.

You ask about our rations. The drawing of them is a fixed fact; every ten days Mrs. B. and I go down with our requisitions, and, now we begin to understand it, you can't know how nicely we live. It takes some dickering, but she is good at that, and we have such a surplus. Of our meat alone (fresh beef) we can always sell seventy-five pounds, and sometimes ninety. A butcher buys it at government price (8½ c.), and pays us cash; this buys butter, eggs, other kinds of meat or "garding sarce;" the milkman takes pork or molasses for his pay; and the baker gives us bread, pound for pound, for our flour. We have pie or cakes now and then, and no more growling; everyone is pleased at the table. We bought some cups and saucers and spoons (we used to have mugs or tin cups and one huge iron spoon put into the sugar), and our table now looks quite like white folks.

I can't help liking Dr. Page, nor do I see who can; he never talks to anyone, but he makes all the reforms we ask for. The patients for the first time get enough to eat, and good food too; and we have only to complain (I mean a just com
plaint) and he rights it.

I have not told you how near I came to going to the front. Miss Dix promised to take me; for a couple of days I got entirely ready and then went in to dress my wounds; I have such a stupid set, I had no one to trust. I set two men to watch for the mail boat; we can see it all the way from Washington. They sat at the windows, and I worked away on those *devilish* Rebs, when, happening to look out, there I saw the boat at our wharf just starting again.

I could have killed the men; but after all it was just as well, for W. was very sick that day and the next, and I had to be with him every moment. I don't know what Miss Dix will say, but I shan't tell her it was stupidity. As W. was so sick, I can say it was he who kept me.

Monday morning (May 18, 1863).

I was interrupted yesterday, and last evening I had to go to church; so, I must hurry up this morning and get this in the post. We have been having such fusses and cross-fits all over the house this morning, about these Rebs, that I feel not at all disposed to write. Some of the nurses are so clever to them, always running and cooking for them, that I've got out of all patience. I say what is good enough for our men is too good for them. Mrs. M. sometimes gets one of hers three breakfasts before he is suited. I wish I had him in my ward; there'd be one hungry man in the house unless he ate what I gave him first. How susceptible some women are to flattery; they (the Rebs) really do have twice the privileges that our Union boys have.

I hope before I write you again we shall have our house filled up once more; I am so tired of this idleness. Those wounded expected yesterday did not come, and we almost despair. I wish the army would move again; but I still believe in Hooker, and expect much from him as soon as the two years men have done going off. I hope you will never notice the nine months' men; they are not worth "shucks." Don't go to the show, will you, when they come home? They just lie round hospitals; this has been full of them, lazier than hounds. All they want is the bounty and to get home. All the Rebs *they* see are the prisoners.

Alexandria (May, 1863).

On Monday morning news came that a boat load of wounded men were on the way for us. They arrived about five o'clock,— such a sick, neglected set as one could ever see; they were some of those who had been in the Rebs hands and had had nothing done for them till they got over the lines,—and then very little, for the accommodations are miserable in those tents. I have no patience at all at so many being kept there; it's such a shame that so little is done for our wounded to get them to comfortable quarters. In every instance, it's been so; a week at least must elapse before anything is done for them. Who does or can control this, I wonder? I got nine for my share, for they had to be distributed all over town. As they are the first wounded that have come for a long time to Alexandria, all are greedy as cormorants to get some.

I expect you will want a full history of mine, so I'll begin at the beginning; and the beginning is that a more wooden, stupid set of dough-heads never lived than my attendants, the whole "biling" being green, nine-months Vermonters. I shall now fully understand "Green Mountain Boys." I never completely realised my loss in all my dear, good boys till that day. I thought I never should get the patients washed and into bed. At last, in despair, I had to press poor W. into the service, though I knew it would bring on fearful excitement and that it would be hours before he could sleep; but he insisted, seeing my despair, on bossing the job, and at last they were comfortably in bed.

Until you could once be in a hospital and see the state of the men as they come in, especially of those who have the blood of three weeks upon them and the dirt of as many months, you can form no idea of the undertaking. But the satisfaction on their faces when all is done and they are finally at rest is very great. Especially when a woman is near to nurse them, they seem so grateful.

These men are all of the Eleventh Corps, and everyone was shot in the first moments of the attack. They are all Germans but one, and he is Irish. I don't believe he ran; he is a spunky little fellow and bears pain "bully." He always smiles when I dress his wound, and only grits his teeth a little when I stuff the lint in. Next to him lies the hero of the ward, a little German boy of seventeen. A piece of shell struck him just by the lower part of the right ear, glancing upward a little, ploughing through the cheek to the bone, and cutting off the end of the nose.

It is almost impossible to give chloroform to patients when the mouth is being operated upon, and he said he did not care for it; so, they performed without any. He never even frowned; the only indication of pain was the shaking of his foot. The room was filled with doctors and lookers-on, and they did nothing but marvel. He can't speak one word of English, is so interesting, and must have been very handsome. The other two in that room are not so badly wounded; only they have been so long neglected that they need much care.

In the next room lies a handsome German with a fractured arm. The next is wounded through the lungs, the ball coming out at the back under the left shoulder. One has a sabre-cut over the head; but it's a flesh wound, and he will soon be right. Next is a boy of seventeen who was shot through the left elbow. But the great case of the house is my "mouth" man, a really noble fellow. He, too, is German, as all the rest. The ball entered just at the point of the collar bone nearest the throat, and lodged in the right shoulder-joint fast and firm, just in the ball of the joint. It was an hour and forty minutes from the time they began to operate upon him till all was done; it's perfectly wonderful how one can live after such an operation, but he is doing splendidly. Worst of all is that my doctor went off Thursday and left me with all these important wounds to take care of, and not a person except these stupid men even to help dress. I have felt so anxious and responsible.

Here I have been writing all this and not telling you one word of the excitement around us. For the last week, all sorts of rumours have been afloat of the invasion of Alexandria; preparations have been making all around, rifle pits dug everywhere, arming negroes, mounting batteries and such things, even the bridge made ready to be destroyed at a moment's notice, and no one permitted to go out of town; but still no one exactly believing, half ridiculing;—till today matters begin to be serious. Rifle pits are dug across all streets leading to the commissary departments, for here lie all the stores for the whole army of the Potomac. Just at the corner of our hospital and just under my window one is dug, and a battery of four guns planted; so, we shall have some shooting (I mean if they come), and since I began to write up comes the orderly, counts out every man in the hospital able to shoulder a gun, and arms them all, so that at a moment's warning they may be ready.

I don't feel the least frightened for myself, but it's horrid to think of these poor wounded fellows and what they would suffer. The town is full of Secesh just waiting for a raid in order to come out openly; and they could fire every hospital at once. I only hope the newspaper reports won't alarm you at home. General Clough, the military governor of this place, was in here tonight, and says the enemy are within ten miles of us, but how strong he doesn't know; of course they are in some force or they would not venture near so many forts as guard this town. Guards are patrolling the streets, and "Halt!" is the continuous cry. I sent a man out for ice tonight, and they snapped him up. I assure you it's very exciting; of course, much is said that is not true, but there must be some cause for all this fuss. I'm so glad my Secesh men are all disposed of. They've been sent to Washington. There are only four in the house now, and those have a guard placed over them tonight. Last night the long roll beat from twelve till two; it sounded good.

I am glad you liked W.'s face; I think it's so good and manly. He begins to look like himself again; his hair has grown out a little, and the wound is entirely healed. Dr. Bellangee scolds me because I closed it so nicely; says it is not half enough of a scar; but his others are bad enough to do him credit. (Dr. Bellangee, assistant surgeon, in charge of Mrs. von Olnhausen's ward; subsequently surgeon-in-chief at Morehead City.) You would have laughed to see him, he was so funny sometimes.

One time he saw some Secesh women passing along; he flew out after them and pulled them by the sleeve: "Here, you Secesh women, you hunting for Rebs? Well, turn to your right and look in the first right-hand door, and there you'll see a bully old Reb"; then he made a profound bow, ran back, hopped into bed, and looked as innocent as if he'd done nothing. They were scared enough, and mad too. Another time he threw his old slippers at two and said, "My new ones are too good for Rebs; they came from Lexington." They excited him so that the doctor forbade their coming through this hall.

I often wish you could see some of the letters I receive from the men when they go away; I sometimes think I'll send them to you. Of course, many of them are poor "or'n'ry" specimens, but they are so earnest, and some of them beautiful in sentiment.

Alexandria (May, 1863).

We have not had any wounded brought from the front yet; but they brought sixteen Rebs from Warrenton (Mosby's men), all shockingly wounded. I had four brought into my ward. I did hate to have them, and felt at first that I could not take care of them; but two were so bad I had to pity them, even after I heard the worst things about one of them. He was a boy only sixteen, so lousy and dirty you could not see his skin, and with long hair, as they all have, like a girl's. He had been fighting but two months, and was an only son. His home is just a little way from here, and his voice was like a child's; and yet when, in the early part of the fight, one of our men had been surprised, had surrendered, and had handed his revolver over to him, the boy shot him dead. It seemed impossible for me to dress his wounds; but his sufferings were so terrible that I forgot for the time how wicked he was. He told me he was sorry he had ever left his home. He wanted so to get well, and kept saying, "Good lady, can't I get a discharge from this hospital? I want to go home."

Poor little fellow! his mother should have kept him there. I saw in another hospital, a few days ago, a little boy only fourteen who had been through all that Peninsular Campaign. How homesick he was, and how tired of soldiering! He was a drummer boy. I believe they have sent him home.

I wish you could see my little turtle; it is not bigger than a cent and is real pretty. Every night it crapples out, and I have such a hunt for him. Yesterday I found him in Mrs. M.'s bed. Then I have a snail that I found at Mt. Vernon last winter; he, too, goes wandering. Every time we are to have a storm he is as big as a quarter-dollar. I keep a pan with wild flowers and roots in it for them to live in, and give them meat and sugar to eat. I always hunt for beetles whenever I go out, and have some live ones. May Day, I spent over the river alone; it is always a pretty sad day to me.

One of my men, who has been to New Jersey on a furlough, says that the Copperheads offered him, if he would desert and stay at home, fifteen dollars a month and house-rent free, and agreed to protect him if our people attempted to arrest him. He was mad, and made such a flaming speech to the crowd that a Union man stepped up and gave him twenty-five dollars for his family, and said if they wanted anything they could come to him. Bully for my man! I wish you could see this river now; every few hours a boat-load of prisoners goes past; today, it is said, three thousand have gone up.

Alexandria (May, 1863).

It is dreadful living so near the field of battle (Chancellorsville). It's only about forty miles from here; and yet you get the real news as soon as we,—I mean, reliable news. From the heights about the town, we can hear the guns, and boats are constantly passing up and down; and yet there are a thousand false to one true rumour. For two days, it was said Hooker had failed and that his loss was fearful; I mean *they* said so, not the papers. I never passed two such days as those were. Then came the good news; and I almost felt that, even if our dear friends are wounded, it was such high honour to be wounded fighting under such a soldier and for such a cause, they were to be envied. Does not this war make one pious, though? I feel like praying all the time. I did not know till now how strong my faith in God and his power was; now I am constantly turning to him. It is useless trying to tell you how I miss my dear friends,—every one gone now except Sergeant G., and he leaves next week. I feel as if I must go, and yet I'm near the front here, and if mine need me I can be with them.

You will think we are always having fusses here,—but such a house! Sunday, when Dr. Page went into Mrs. B.'s store-room she asked him for some things that the men in the dispensary had refused to give up, but that had been sent to her by the Sanitary Commission. Dr. Page told her he thought the dispensary was the proper place for them, and that, furthermore, he meant to confiscate everything sent to the nurses in the way of delicacies or clothes. You may bet my back was up; so yesterday morning I went to him and asked if he was in earnest; he said, "Yes." I told him that rather than give what things I had to those miserable, drinking boys, I'd throw them from the windows.

"Do they drink?"

"Doctor, you know they do, when you look in their faces. My friends send those things for soldiers, not for clerks and stewards who, I know, constantly invite their friends and treat them to delicacies and wines."

"Are you sure?"

"Yes, within a week."

So, I explained what I knew; also, that they had used a large quantity of choice stores left with them, subject to my particular order only, by a Philadelphia lady who was not permitted to bring them upstairs. I had never had but two orders filled, and then all was gone. I told him, moreover, that I thought it was wrong to place so much temptation before mere boys.

"I agree with you," he said; "and now, when I will take all the wines and liquors from the dispensary, will you take charge of and deliver them?"

I told him I thought there were others better qualified than I (meaning Mrs. B.). "Ha! you come with complaints and then shirk responsibility!"

So, I accepted at once rather than be charged that way; but I went right to the chaplain and told him he must go and beg Dr. Page to put Mrs. B. in my place; it was so wrong to take it from her. I knew she would feel hurt, told him I was a dough-head, and that he must say so. He talked the doctor over, and now she is to have them.

Alexandria, Sunday (June, 1863).

You must have been surprised at my letter announcing W.'s return so soon after his leaving. I was so stunned at seeing him I don't know what I wrote about him. Anyway, I knew nothing of his wound or what he had gone through to get here until after that; so, I have no fear of giving a twice-told tale. You can form no idea how utterly prostrated he was with fatigue and loss of blood and the shock of the ball. From Monday morning, at three, till about eight on Sunday morning, when he was wounded, the regiment was marching and fighting all the time. In fording the Rapidan the water was up to their armpits; they charged on a body of about one hundred and fifty Rebs (I think he said), who were building a most substantial bridge across the river, and took them all prisoners. He said the boys were just as full of fun as if they had waded in for play; when they saw a Reb hiding or skulking off, they would call, "Come here, Johnny Reb" (they all call them that name), "we won't hurt you." It was about four o'clock, they were all wet through, the night was cold, not a fire was allowed, and they just bivouacked in the woods without any cover. What these poor souls have to suffer!

When W. first fell, all supposed he was killed; he was insensible. When he came to, G. and M.—another noble fellow—were kneeling beside him, tears rolling down their cheeks. They had only time to say goodbye and receive his messages when they had to leave him. After they had exhausted their ammunition (he had fired forty rounds before he fell), they were ordered to the rear to replenish, and bore him along so tenderly, saw him cared for at a hospital, and went to the front again. He doesn't know how long he stayed there; but before night the hospital was shelled, and he only remembers hobbling up. He must have got to another hospital, as, early in the morning, that was shelled, and again all were started off somewhere else.

He took the road to Falmouth with the one idea to get back to Dr. Bellangee and myself. He walked some time; then a negro came along, took him into his wagon and drew him some four miles; the driver's road was then another way, so he laid him down to wait again. Soon a white man with a government wagon came along, but refused to take him up. W. threatened him, when the man got down and lifted him in. He says the horror of that ride can't be told; the man drove so frightfully over such an awful road. At last he reached a hospital in Falmouth; as he lay there quite exhausted, he heard someone say, "The cars leave in half an hour for Aquia Creek."

He inquired the way to the station, and only remembers getting on the platform when the cars started. Then he only knows he passed the night in a hospital there, and someone gave him his bed. All this time he had eaten nothing (and in fact since they had started on that Monday morning he had never eaten the three days rations in his haversack). Again, someone said near him, "The boat leaves directly for Washington." He asked if he could not go; they told him, not without a permit from the provost-marshal, and there was no time for that; so, he remembers stealing out in the rear, to avoid the guards, and coming down to the wharf. Just as he crossed the plank, it was taken in and the boat started. This was about four. He remembers nothing again until he was at the wharf, sometime in the night, at Washington, lying on the floor, so cold, and begging someone to close the doors.

Next morning, he went up to the Sanitary rooms near there, had his wound dressed for the first time,—he thinks with camphor, by some fussy old woman who "deared" him and, though so miserable, made him laugh, she "poor-thinged" him so. He then asked to be sent to Alexandria; again, they told him he must first go to the provost-marshal, and that his office was two miles off. He knew he could not get there, so he inquired the way to the Alexandria wharf. All this time seems just like a dream to him; he said he was conscious of no pain or of any other thought, except "When I get there it will be all right." He walked half a mile to the wharf; they refused to take him, but said perhaps the government tugs would, and they lay back where he started from; so back the dear soul struggled again.

Isn't it pitiful? He just asked a tug if they stopped at Alexandria, and they told him yes (so strange all this time nobody questioned him, when usually one can't stir without a challenge). He walked on board, sat down in the coal hole, and remembered nothing more till he was walking up the stairs here.

Dr. Bellangee and I were both sitting down after having dressed the wounds, hearing the news read; the papers had just been brought in when he opened the door. I saw this poor, dusty fellow all covered with powder and blood, all bent, leaning on a stick and looking so old; I never dreamed it was W., nor did any one, till he said, "Well, they've plugged me again." We all rushed round him, and everyone burst into tears,—even the doctor could not command himself. W. just fell on the nearest bed, and the tears gushed out.

He said so piteously, "I'm here at last." I can't tell you what we felt. In a moment the room was full,—clerks, doctors, everybody who could hobble came in. His eyes looked frightfully dilated and staring, and he was frothing at the mouth as if crazy. After we recovered a little from our shock the doctor took him to a room by himself, examined his wound, and forbade his speaking or being spoken to, even by me. The room was made perfectly dark, and there the dear fellow has lain ever since, just between life and death. Yesterday noon his eyes contracted, and he began to show symptoms more favourable.

Dr. B. says he cannot understand how he ever got here in the state he was in; he never knew such an instance of will overcoming bodily suffering. He thinks now the skull is not fractured; only that the brain is shocked, and that with careful nursing he will soon be well. You can judge a little how weak he is, as he is allowed only one cracker and a tumbler of milk a day. It is a frightful responsibility, for the doctor says it all depends on me now; that one overfeeding will kill him. I have written you a long chapter on W.; but he is our only wounded one yet from the grand fight. You will be surprised we are so; every moment we have been expecting the wounded, but all the boats go by to Washington. I'm so sorry; I long to have them to care for; but I won't begin to make comments. I am so harassed by the thousand rumours, I mean to hear or believe nothing till I know for certain.

I think I told you about the fuss we had with Dr. Page, H., etc.,

about some things the Sanitary Committee sent to Mrs. B.,—
an elegant lot for the expected wounded. When she at last got
them, those miserable toads had eaten and drank everything but
twelve cans of milk. Twenty-five pounds of sugar, twelve bottles
of pickles, twelve bottles of cordial, and some other things had
all been confiscated by them for their own use. Isn't it a shame?
Just look how the people at home are cheated and duped! I
wonder anybody there ever trusts any one concerned in the
war.

Chapter 5

As already stated, in July of 1863 Mrs. von Olnhausen was furloughed because of illness. Returning to Lexington for a month or more, in September she again reported for duty. A few pages (the last she wrote) of her *Autobiography* will best sum up this period and the changes in her duties which it brought about. The letters which follow the *Autobiography* cover her experiences during the remaining months of 1863 in a new field of work,—the just established hospital at Morehead City, North Carolina.

Although it is unsafe to criticise without full knowledge of the facts and conditions, it would seem to have been more appropriate to send a woman of such enthusiasm for surgical nursing, of such personal courage, and of such physical vigour, to the front rather than to a hospital then so remote from hostilities, and in which medical cases were almost certain to preponderate. Mrs. von Olnhausen always was restive in Morehead City, and never was persuaded that she might not have done far more for the soldiers had she been sent to a field hospital, or at least to one close to the seat of war, where she could have devoted herself wholly to the care of severe wounds and capital operations. Miss Dix was doubtless greatly influenced by the wishes of Dr. Bellangee, who naturally desired to retain so reliable a nurse and so devoted a friend in this Morehead hospital, which he himself had organised.

(FROM THE *AUTOBIOGRAPHY*)

There was at this time an epidemic of dysentery all through the hospital, and at last I was taken sick with it, and remained many days half conscious. All the nurses declared they were too busy to attend to me, so I lay alone most of the time. In the meantime, the house surgeon attended me very carefully, and ordered a convalescent to sit in the room and supply my wants. He was the funniest little man I ever saw,—a shoe-maker who got a big bounty as substitute, but whose legs were so short that he kept falling out of the ranks. He finally got sick, and was sent here. He had big, round blue eyes, and in my half-delirium they looked as large as a cup. He was a German, and never took those eyes off me. He sat by the door from morning till night, never moving except to eat his meals. At last my friends came, and as soon as I could be moved I was taken home on leave of absence.

After all the turmoil of that life it was so delightful to be quiet; but I soon began to recover, and in a month started back to Alexandria. When I got there, everything seemed different, as most of the nurses had been discharged and nearly all the doctors changed. I found two letters awaiting me. One was from my old house surgeon, Dr. S., asking me to come to him at Chattanooga and take charge of a large hospital with a friend of mine. The other was from my old ward surgeon, Dr. Bellangee, who was now in charge of a large hospital at Morehead City, N. C, asking me, and also the same friend, to come there. We decided to take the latter place.

We had a tiresome passage from New York to New Berne, and were glad to get on shore. New Berne seemed pleasant, and I would gladly have stayed there; but Dr. Bellangee was waiting to take us at once to Morehead City, where his hospital was established. He had done wonders in the short time he had been there. Eight barracks had been built, each containing about seventy-five beds, some of them already fitted up. This was certainly the best hospital I saw in the war. We had an excellent steward who provided most liberally, and we had everything the sick and wounded could ask for. Dr. Bellangee was a martinet about the hospital, seeming to be always everywhere. His skill in surgery was wonderful, and his care unceasing.

Morehead "City" was made up of about ten houses, and was the terminus of the railroad, so transportation for the wounded from New Berne was easy. There were at first very few patients, and I feared we should have too little work; but they began to send us patients from the over-filled hospitals in New Berne, and there were some skirmishes between the pickets around us, so we soon had no cause to complain. At first, we had an assistant surgeon (so called) who was very tenacious of his rights, and once threatened me with discharge because in the middle of the night I applied a mustard draft, without consulting him, to a man who had colic. He said it was a surgical operation, and that I had no business to perform it. Dr. Bellangee, when complained to next morning, laughed quietly, wrote out a permission for me to use mustard if very necessary, read it to the surgeon, and sent it to me by his orderly. After that I could have covered the men with plaisters if I had chosen.

After the corruption and constant fusses of the Mansion House, ruled by unscrupulous cooks and a more unscrupulous steward, one can't describe the peace of this hospital. One thing was rather strange in Morehead City; not until the last few months of the war did the Sanitary Commission ever reach us. It was impossible to get any liquors or any delicacies except such as were sent me from Lexington. Those friends, I am thankful to say, never failed me. I am sure none of the men who knew me will ever forget Lexington, though they will have long ago forgotten me, for my foreign name was too hard to remember. I was always called Madam, or Mrs. O., or Mrs. Von; sometimes they twisted the O into all sorts of words. My little Reb, when he wrote me, called me "dear Mrs. Woe," and some have written to the care of the Lexington Post-Office, directed to Mrs. Zaugh or Mrs. Owe.

It was singular how one could detect the nationality of a man, however poor English he might speak, by the way he bore suffering. Our men (I mean Americans) were impressible; the moment they were housed they were so cheerful and determined to get well that they usually did from sheer grit, however badly wounded. The Germans, though equally plucky in bearing pain, lay back with such a resigned manner, a sort of "As God wills" air. An Irishman complained of everything, and a Frenchman was the hardest to please of all; he was always worse hurt and more wounded than any other.

Our Yankees were always ready to help and amuse others when themselves suffering ever so much, and it was everywhere remarked how much more quickly they got well. The poor Rebels were so discontented at finding themselves prisoners and wounded, and had been so badly fed, that their wounds were the hardest of all to heal, and it was some time before one could make them hopeful for the future. They believed, too, that if cured they would be sent to Northern prisons and treated as our men had been by them. While in the ward I treated and tended all alike, much to the disgust of some who looked on.

★★★★★★

In view of some of the references to her Secession patients in Mrs. von Olnhausen's earlier letters, it may seem that this last statement is rather too complacent. Her friends, however, will appreciate that however she might rail at these Rebels, her humanity was too deep to permit of her neglecting them in the slightest degree.

The following letter, descriptive of her return journey to Washington, shows how ready she was to extract entertainment from the most untoward circumstances.

Alexandria, Sept. 4, 63, Friday.

I arrived here yesterday morning. Had time in Washington to fly to Miss Dix and report, and get the boat; and thought I should write at once; but Mrs. B. wanted me to go right back to Washington with her, so I was too tired when I got home to think of anything; but I will begin at the beginning.

All F's notes and telegrams did not one bit of good. I had a lonely ride from Boston to the (Fall River) boat; but the last part of the route a pleasant woman from Ohio sat with me and offered her husband's services. I told her, however, the conductor would attend to me. He went on board and was most polite, but could not find F's friend; so, I went into the cabin, and that's the last I saw of anybody. I waited till nine before I gave up. I don't know how many times I sent, and finally word came that all state-rooms had been engaged for two weeks to come; so, then I began to hunt for a sleeping place.

By great persuasion I got one on the floor, close by the gang way. Such a crowd you never saw. One hundred and fifty women and babies got on at Newport, and everyone was sick; the sea was very rough, and even the poor little babies were as sick as their mothers. One woman, a lady, too, had five children, one a baby; they all were so sick, she just laid the baby on the floor and left it. I took it up and held it till it slept, and then laid it on the foot of someone's bed. You never saw such a sight; everyone who came in or out stepped over me.

We had such a jolly old stewardess. A waiter from upstairs came down in the middle of the night and wanted Mrs. F.; said that her husband was sick as death, and she must come right away. The stewardess called out for Mrs. F.; nobody answered. "How can I find her?" she said.

He went and came back, saying, "Mr. F. says you can find her in a berth in the back part; you will know her by a great pimple she has. I disremember where he said it was."

"How can I find out Mrs. F. and her pimple? You go back and tell Mr. F. if he wants Mrs. F. and her pimple he can come and hunt her up; I've got business enough of my own to attend to." The man went off, and just then Mrs. F. appeared in full undress, very sick, and tugging a very sick baby. Stewardess and I were glad to have our curiosity relieved with regard to the whereabouts of that pimple; it was on one side of her forehead and might modestly be called a horn, it stuck out so far. She sent word to Mr. F. that she and baby were too sick to live, and he must come right to her. No Mr. F. appeared, and she and her pimple retired for the night.

Another woman kept calling, "Oh, stewardess, do come help me, I am so sea-sick."

She was flying around making beds, and said, "Everyone must do their own sea-sickness; I've got a hundred and fifty beds to make, and that's as much as I can do without doing your sea-sickness."

Four women were sitting together, and all so sick; she brought one basin and said, "There, you must all be sick in that, I have not half enough to go round." Altogether, it was a very funny night.

We were delayed by the fog, and it was eight before we got in. I gave my checks to the express man, and then had to wait till eleven before I could get my trunks. The ride to and through Philadelphia was as dreary as anything could well be. I sat beside a copperhead who made me furious, so I tried to go to sleep. I think the horse-car arrangement through Philadelphia is too mean for anything. I never was so sleepy and so cold.

At twelve I got into the night car, and might have had a good sleep except for an English cockney girl who "set up for shapes" and couldn't go to bed because a man was sleeping in the same car.

"Mama, 'ow can I go to bed when there is a man here?"

"Well, dear, he has a right here."

"But, Mama, what 'orrid customs! You see, ladies, I have only just crossed the water, and it's so 'ard to get used to the customs, we think it's so hawful to sleep with a man in the room."

It turned out afterwards she had lived here all her life and had been to England only on a visit. The man lay and laughed loud as he could. She opened her sack and asked Mama "which wine she would 'ave, port or sherry." She took a big horn, and then regularly undressed, for all her scruples, right in the alley, and finally looked into this man's berth and said, "'Ow can you sleep with the curtains so close, no hair? I must have mine open and the port side door too;" at first she had insisted on pinning his together herself. All this while a funny man was, with many inducements, persuading her to sleep in the car; her modesty seemed to vanish with him. She talked for two hours, and then my bunk broke down and I came near mashing her to death; the fright silenced her, and I got another bunk and finally slept. Miss Dix was glad to see me, and is decidedly of the opinion that I must go to New Berne. I have seen a plan of the hospital and it is splendid there, with many wounded men who need a surgical nurse; but when I got here Dr. Page was so glad to see me, and said he wanted me so much that I don't know what to do. I shall let Miss Dix decide when she comes this afternoon. The Mansion House is dreary enough; I don't believe I can stay here.

We have got into a fine scrape with our mess. H. (we think it was he) has sued the butcher (I mean Government, through his information) and fined him (the butcher) fifty dollars, which he had to pay. Of course, Mrs. B. appealed, and the trial has been going on for a week, till today it's decided against us. Now we have fifty dollars to pay and, besides, lose thirty dollars' worth of meat which they have confiscated because, owing to the fuss, it was left over till this month. All the nurses except Mrs. W. and us two refuse to pay their part; so we do it alone. Mrs. B. has advanced me the money till pay-day comes.

Miss Dix says she will take it to higher authority, and Dr. Page says that after we had drawn the meat, we had a right to do what we liked with it. I know there is no right or justice in it; but what are we to do? So now we are back on bread and beef; the only thing is we have enough of these; but, oh, it's hard living after home fare. There can never be an end to fusses in the Mansion House.

Transport Ship, Pier 12,
New York, Tuesday (September 8, 1863).

Were I to write all my adventures since my last letter to you, I would have to write a longer one than you would care to read.

I saw Miss Dix after I wrote, and she decided I must go to New Berne anyway; so, I had to tell Dr. Page. I hated to tell him and the chaplain, for they have both been such good friends to me. Dr. Page asked me to stay; but I told him it was impossible; I could not remain where H. (the steward) was. Then he asked me would I come back to him when he had a hospital without H. He wanted me to promise that I would; so, I did, and the last thing he said at parting was that I must keep my promise. After I went out, Dr. B. reports that he said, "There goes the best and truest woman I've met in the service; I like every inch of her." Miss Dix said we would have to leave about Wednesday; so, Saturday I went to Washington to see Mr. U., the beetle man. I did all my packing that evening, and Sunday, at three, we left the Mansion House, for a while I hope. But now hear the worst of it! Just as we were getting into the ambulance came an order for our arrest and search! There's a sister for you! That devil H. sent information to Dr. Page, who was out of town, that we were removing large quantities of hospital stores, and so he ordered the officer of the day to arrest, etc.! Dr. Barnes happened to be the man. He came right to Mrs. B. and told her that rather than do it he would be "broke of the service."

He sent off for the chaplain, who came in furious. Now the only stores we took with us at all were a box he gave us, which had for a long time stood in the store-room, but had never been unpacked, and those things I brought from home. I found it would cost too much to bring anything more. Mrs. B. did not tell me, so I did not understand at all the fuss. If I had I never would have left so. I would have insisted on an examination and have brought H. to grief. The first I knew of it was when we were half-way to Baltimore. I don't blame Dr. Page at all. Mrs. B. is furious with him; but of course, he knew nothing of the truth, and had to act as he did. I am prepared for anything now! All the clerks and stewards were around to see the fun, and must have been much disappointed.

Such a ride to Washington as we had was never known; the road was crowded with soldiers and horses, everything moving,—all showing a battle is soon to come, I think. The dust was so thick we had to stop for it, and some of the horses even fell down the embankments. Then came up a frightful storm and nearly drowned us. When we got to Washington there was no sleeping-car, not even a hook to hang our things on. It was such a long, sleepy ride, ending in that horrid horse-car arrangement through Philadelphia. It was very early morning when we got here, and we could not see the proper authorities till ten, so we went "bumming" around to find a breakfast. How forlorn a city is early in the morning.

The captain said we might come on board tonight, though he should not sail till some time tomorrow. So, we came with our traps this evening. Could you see us! Such a dirty vessel, a half-and-half, sometimes steams and sometimes sails,—both poorly, I guess. I wish you could see the cockroaches, too; there never was the like before, I think; everything is covered with them, and everything black with smoke. I think, too, everyone is drunk on board; which does not make it any too comfortable. When one goes nursing, all things must be expected. The captain says if the weather is good we shall be there in three days. I am glad to go to sea at last, but somehow, I feel so strange; I seem to be drifting about without any will of my own. Miss S. would have a nice chance to talk "Heavenly Fatherish"!

New Berne, N. C., Sunday evening
(September 13, 1863).

(Spelling adopted in official reports; but elsewhere one finds also Newberne and Newbern.)

We are so far safe on our journey, as you will be glad to learn. We have still thirty miles farther to go, and shall then, I hope, find friends and a comfortable home for a while at least. Dr. Bellangee's hospital is at Morehead City, instead of here, and it's been such a bother to get things straightened out. We leave here in the morning at nine, so in my next I shall be able to tell you all about it. That night I wrote you from New York I did not dare tell you how homesick I already felt. I think you would have been hardly willing for me to go if you could have seen me in that dirty, miserable ship. I did not dare think of home, or that it was only a week since I had left you all; it seemed a month by that time.

I can't describe that ship, no words can; if there was one redeeming thing about it, I would tell it. It was owned by Jersey people; everyone from cook up was hail-fellow, nobody saw to anything, the cabin was never cleaned while we were on board, and as to the other places, you can have no idea of the filth. How I ever could be brought to sleep in that berth amazes me now; it was frightful. Of course, I passed all my time, except the few hours I *did* sleep, entirely alone on deck; for Mrs. B. was sick from the time we started, and nobody was even civil. There were lots of officers on board, everybody drank, and all were sick a good part of the way, except Colonel C. and myself. The first night was pretty frightful; the old tub rolled badly enough. We were about thirty miles below Navesink lights when a storm came on, and the captain had to run back to Sandy Hook, where we lay till next day at ten. My! weren't the people sick!

Yesterday morning we got to Cape Hatteras, where we lay all day. I went ashore in the tug and wandered about as I liked. There are two forts there, garrisoned with North Carolina troops; they don't look like our Northern soldiers; but such a beach and such waves I never saw,—miles of it, and the breakers are fearful. The beach, though so beautiful, is very dangerous, being full of quicksands. At noon Ensign Livermore of the gunboat stationed there came with his gig and invited Mrs. B. and me to dine with him; he is a Massachusetts man and was most polite. The captain of the tug, too, invited us to dine with him; so, we had no lack of attention.

The fact is women are so scarce they are appreciated. Then, I expect, on the ship the men were mostly young and thought we were two old cats and of no account; but since I came ashore I find they all thought I was Secesh and going over the lines. I remember two or three asked me if I was. I answered no; but as B. used to say, "did not feel like talking," so did not enlighten them. I would have been furious if I had thought they took me for a Reb. We got in here this morning by daylight. It is such a lovely town,—not the streets or houses, I mean,—but the trees, every street so beautifully shaded, and with such large gardens. I wanted to go to the fort, but a big rain came, so we have had to stay in. I shall be glad when we are quiet and settled; a fortnight of rushing around is as much as I want at a time.

Morehead City, N. C., September 24, 1863.
I can't tell exactly what my impression was in getting here; it looked forlorn enough. We are thirty miles from New Berne,

cars once a day. Dr. Bellangee received us most kindly; at once took us over the grounds, but did not give us our places for a couple of days, most of which time I spent in the woods about us. The open sea is only two miles away, and the air is splendid; enough of it, too, for it blows a tempest. All is in such an unfinished state yet here; but doctor is driving the men to get them on. Six of the large barracks (forty-five beds each) are completed, three or four more are to be soon done. They are not all filled yet, but there is some talk of breaking up the New Berne hospitals and sending all the sick here, which I should think would be done, it's so unhealthful there.

We have only two hundred yet here; most all are Massachusetts men,—the Seventeenth, Twenty-Third, and Twenty-Fifth; and two or three more lie all around here; the Twenty-eighth, too, is in New Berne. It seems good to have Massachusetts men sick; but most all are too well to be interesting. Night before last, about one, a train came down express; next morning I was told that the Second Massachusetts had come to garrison a fort near here. I tell you it made my heart beat; but I soon found it was the Second Artillery. It's only been from home five weeks, and already so many are sick with chills. I have three of them very ill with fever.

I told you I was too mad last Sunday to write; the reason was we had planned to go on a little excursion,—all the mess; but the chaplain made a fuss and stopped it, and asked us as a favour to go to church, at three. That was bad enough; but after we were done there, and thoroughly shrived, Dr. Bellangee stood up and said he would excuse no one, and expected us all to follow him and go to dress parade of the Eighty-Sixth (I believe), that lies near us, and after that attend services there. I asked to be excused, but he said no.

You may think I was mad; here we were marched out like so many cats,—first the two doctors (doctor has only one assistant); then the steward; after them we two; and after us all the lame, halt, and blind by twos over this sand for a quarter of a mile to see the poorest drilling I ever saw and hear the worst preaching. I got so thoroughly cross that I could have sworn every moment. To crown all he would not then excuse us, but made us all march back again. I would not speak another word the whole evening. Did you ever get that mad you would not be satisfied? That's the way I was; I could not even sleep.

Morehead City, September 28 (1863).

I was so glad to get your letter yesterday, and should have answered it immediately, but was sick in bed. I can't know the cause, for I'm sure it could not be too much eating, as in all our poor eating this beats all. I don't mean in quantity, for I never was in a hospital so liberally fed; but as I can't eat salt horse, and never did like potatoes and onions, and, until this week, we have had to buy all our bread, which has been both sour and heavy, I don't think it was eating that did it. I felt weak as a rat yesterday, but am all right again, and such a beautiful day never was seen.

We had a very bad storm last night and looked out for wrecks this morning, but can see none. The surf sounds so grand, and it's just like a June day. So many mocking-birds are singing, and, as we have had no frost yet, it's beautifully green in the woods. I believe I begin to feel a little less homesick, but am no better contented with my work, and have fully determined not to stay here long. As far as the doctor goes, I could not ask better; he is kind as can be, and gives us every privilege; but I really have nothing to do. I should die to have so little work; I don't believe in wasting time so. I am sure I'm equal to better things. I certainly did not come into the service to play; and every walk I take I feel as if I were a real humbug. I have only one man really sick, and those I've had never stay sick more than three or four days; as soon as they breathe this fine air they get right up.

Morehead City, November 12 (1863).

Mansfield Hospital.

I first of all must ask forgiveness for neglecting so long to write; but you see I every day expected Miss Dix's answer, and then, though it came three or four days ago, I felt so disappointed at its not containing an immediate recall that it put me out of heart for writing. Excuses over, I'll tell about Miss Dix's brief letter,—same old style: "My child, be patient; not one nurse in any hospital has much to do just now, but you'll soon have enough to do. I may send you to Nashville or Hilton Head, circumstances will determine which! In the meantime, do not leave without authority!" So, I wait! Don't think I shall leave here without regret, for really, I never have had so many friends in any place.

This climate is beautiful; only one frost yet, night before last, and that slight; and the sea always so grand, and making it so healthful. Then these boat excursions are too jolly; always some adventure. Getting aground and having to wait for hours for the tide is a common experience. The people, too, are such a different race from any I've ever met before; they beat Illinois hollow. Here they sit from morning till night in their cabins, with their snuff sticks, chewing, chewing, never reading; sometimes spinning or knitting a little; looking so vacant; living on fish and "Eupon" tea.

I don't know how the word is spelled, but it sounds like that; it's an evergreen something like myrtle; they parch the leaves and then boil them. To me it tastes like senna. They have very little flour and less cornmeal; but the everlasting sweet potatoes are everywhere. Such a life! You can't make them talk. There they sit and chew or pipe. They need us. This Shackelford Island opposite us is I don't know how many miles long. It's very narrow, never half a mile wide. The best house on it an Irishman would be ashamed of. They are all fishermen, and it's said there is not a Reb on the whole island.

I am going to give a picture of one of my days and then I'll have done. I rise at *reveille* (six). I never go into the ward before breakfast, so I have time to bathe and dress at my ease. Breakfast about seven. From there I go to the cook house to see what the bill of fare is for the day; then over here in time for the surgeon's call at eight. I go all around with the doctor, do what I have to do in this ward (Division 1); then, at nine, doctor and I go to Division 7, a big ward for commissioned officers I have charge of. I stay another hour there, then over to the cook house, make my puddings, back to Division 1 in time for the mail at eleven, over to the cook-house to see that I get the best that is going for my trays, back again to my wards to see dinner distributed, then off to my dinner in another direction.

After dinner, I pass an hour or two in this ward (here are all the sickest men), unless we go for a walk. At four I go to the cook-house again to see about supper, canter back to give it to them, then canter off to supper. Evenings I generally pass with Mrs. B. Tattoo at eight; but we don't have to mind that; ten is our hour for breaking up. So, you can see what every day is when we are not off sailing. All this cantering round is very healthy, as you must know. I'm always in the open air.

I send you this little rough sketch of our hospital grounds, so you can see where I live. It is quite a walk to the different places I have to visit through the day. These large barrack wards each have forty beds and can hold more. Just now there is hardly an empty bed in the whole hospital, but there are no sick men except in Division 1, and these have only chronic diarrhoea; just have to have their diet regulated and to lie in bed; they need no other care.

Morehead City, December 10 (1863).
Still here! How much longer I'm to write from this I don't know; and there are thousands now who need me. I feel so discouraged. I have a mind to cut Miss Dix altogether and run away; you can't know how impatient I feel. She told me in her last brieflet to wait with patience till the sixth, and then she should write again and assign me to another place. That is why I did not write Sunday; I wanted to await her letter. It has not come, and I'm mad as a pig. Really you can't know how I want to get out of this.

Yesterday they brought me a wounded Rebel, not wounded by fighting, but in making shingles or something. He cut his hand fearfully, and the artery was entirely severed; it keeps bleeding, so he has to be watched day and night. It's pretty tedious to have to sit all day looking at the very dirtiest paw you ever saw. He is so frightened about himself. This and the nigger who was shot, all for love, are the only wounds I've had to dress, so I am forgetting all I knew.

Morehead City, December (1863).
The whole hospital has been in such a state of consternation and trustification the last ten days it's been impossible to write or do anything one ought to. News came at that time that this hospital was to be broken up and all scattered to the winds. Nobody knew for why, only that it was to be done. I was sure then of leaving, expecting perhaps to have to go home, when Miss Dix did not order me somewhere; but Thursday night, about six, the inspectors arrived. We were not expecting them, and had made no preparations. Dr. Bellangee suggested waiting till daylight; but they thought to catch us, and started about eight

with lanterns, blundering round, waking up the sick men, and poking into everything. There were six of them.

Next morning, they started early, without Dr. Bellangee, and went over all again. When they left the doctor, they said it was inevitable that the hospital be closed; the orders were peremptory from General Butler (who had never seen the house anyway). When they got back to headquarters, Dr. McC. said "he was —— if it should be closed; it was the best regulated hospital he ever saw,—everything was as near perfect as could be." Dr. Bellangee was radiant, for he did not know where they would send him to, and was so nicely fixed here. The weather is beautiful, like spring; we still go boating and rowing.

Chapter 6

Despite her continued pleadings to be sent to the front, Mary von Olnhausen remained at Morehead City throughout the greater part of 1864. Her impatience at inaction was very great during the early months of that year; but the numbers of sick and wounded gradually increased; a large influx of refugee "poor whites" gave scope for her extraordinary loving- kindness; and, in the fall, came an enemy worse than the Rebels—yellow fever—for her to do battle with, especially in trying to rescue from its grim clutches her beloved Dr. Bellangee.

Her devotion and skill could not, however, save him; and soon after his death, worn out in body and mind, she herself contracted the disease and lay for many days critically ill. Her care for others was requited by the tender nursing which at this time she herself received; and as soon as it was possible she was taken North to that Lexington which she always looked upon as her haven of refuge. The following letters cover these nine months of impatience, of ever-increasing work and responsibility, and, finally, of the great sorrow which came in the death of her dear chief.

> January 1 (1864), 12 a. m., Friday morning.
> Happy New Year, and many kisses to all at home!
> I was going to have such a good time writing and watching the Old Year out, as I have done for many years, and singing my one hymn, when, just as I had got a letter written to C., came in Captain C., wet through to the skin, cold as the iciest of ice, hungry like a wolf, and, more than all, with a badly sprained ankle (I'm hanged if I know how to spell that last word—is it *k* or *c*?). Of course, I had to leave all and attend to him, and so at twelve, instead of having written you a good, cheerful letter, as I should have done, I was *suaging* (N. C. dialect) his swollen limb (can't venture that other word again), and only had time

to begin this and sing my *hime.*

Now today I'm all down in the bluest depths, cross or something, and impatient, forgetting in my wilful wickedness that the good God has given me anything this past year to be thankful for, even in this sterile spot, and only remembering friends and joys that I can't reach, and looking gloomily backward instead of hopefully and joy fully forward as a good, pious Christian ought to do and does.

I'm sure I would be pious if I could, but I've tried and tried and can't catch the spirit; either I don't know how, or the Lord won't help me; "I'se so wicked, pears like." Anyway, I'm not always so desponding, thank fortune, and am sometimes singing praises all day long. Good Lord, deliver me from this slough; I'm in it fairly up to the chin.

To read the following letter, and to remember that the writer of it was then nearly fifty years old, is to gain some idea of the abounding energy of this "second-best *belle.*"

Morehead City (as usual), January 3, 1864.
I am so discouraged about writing, I have no heart to. First of all, now let me darn my commander-in-chief. Here she will keep me for the rest of my life, I suppose. She wrote to Dr. Bellangee to ask if he was satisfied with his nurses and could make them useful. Dr. B. of course wrote, yes; and so I'm to remain. I feel so disheartened, I can't get over it. To be sure, just now we have two very bad typhoid cases; but they can't last much longer, and then I shall be out of a job and can just loaf. For the last fortnight, I have had a ward cram-full; but everyone is up for discharge or furlough, and there are no more sick here; so then what'll I do? Why can't somebody want me and make me come?

You will be surprised to know I went to a real ball New Year's night. All sorts of fine doings over at Fort Macon. Dr. Bellangee would not take a denial from Mrs. B. or me; so, we had to go, though I really had nothing to wear. I patched up that purple skirt of mine, and the white waist that D. gave me; but I had no gloves or boots, only thick ones, and felt rather shabby; and then having hardly a spear of hair! I was not first-best, but, as there were only seven ladies, I had to be a *belle,* and so danced continuously.

You can have no idea of the storm that night; it never rained harder. The sea was fearful. We went a mile to the station on a hand car, and then took the tug to the fort (two miles); it was about as wild a night as one would care to put to sea in; and just after we arrived there came up the awfulest thunder-shower you ever heard; it sounded as if all the guns in the fort were exploding. Our party of five ladies was the only one that ventured out. There were thirty-seven invited (ladies, I mean) and they had made big preparations. The dance-hall was trimmed with flags and evergreens, the music was good, and the supper fine; but it was the dullest affair I ever went to.

All were so disappointed that it was impossible to get up any life. It was so stormy we could not leave till five in the morning; and then when we got to the station the mule who dragged our hand car down had run away, and the *nigs* had run away too; so, we had to come that mile on our tired pedals. It was a tough walk with the gale dead ahead, and nearly blowing us off the track into the sea; for it is only a pier that the cars run on. I flattered myself I'd have an hour's sleep anyway; but just as I got upstairs they came and said F. was worse. As soon as I looked at him I saw he wouldn't live long, so just hurried off my ball fixings and stayed with him till he died, about nine that morning.

Morehead City, January 19 (1864).

I have only a few minutes just to tell you how tired I am and let you know where I am. For the past ten days, I have had no attendant but one Frenchman, who does not speak a word of English. When this last call was made for all able-bodied men to return to their regiments, my watchman had to go; and the same day both my attendants (of course, broken-down invalids) were taken sick, one with typhoid and one with acute dysentery, so I had to watch all day and part of every night, besides doing extra cooking and all kinds of work through the day. Of course, I am tired out; as you may see when I say I have fourteen patients all in bed, ten with the worst kind of typhoid pneumonia, so they have to be lifted and fed and washed, as they can't raise a hand. I have not left my ward, except to eat, since I wrote last.

Morehead City, February 5, 1864.

I wrote you on Monday that news had come that New Berne

was attacked. On Tuesday, about twelve o'clock, a despatch came that Newport Barracks, ten miles from this, was attacked by a large Rebel force. It was held by the Ninth Vermont, one company of the Second Massachusetts Heavy Artillery, and a single company of the Nineteenth Wisconsin. Colonel Jourdan of the One Hundred and Fifty-Eighth New York started from here immediately with what few men he had left (the best had already been sent in defence of New Berne), and two field-pieces and a few men from Company C of the Massachusetts H. A., leaving this place almost defenceless. I forgot to say that all the night before the cars were running, bringing down arms and ammunition for the recruits of the One Hundred and Fifty-Eighth and Second; until they were brought there was not a single gun left in the town; *smart*, I think.

Well, to go on with my story. Jourdan started with his raw recruits, but the cars were attacked and he had to come back. Soon the negroes began to flock in; they came by hundreds, such frightened beings, leaving everything except their children behind them. The gunboats (one, I mean, a small one) came up and lay opposite the town. Every citizen was compelled to take arms, and every negro was put to work on the entrenchments. Such a scurrying time you never saw. All the company stores were sent on board the ships, and all the stores of the regiment too; and every one began to pack his traps. Everything seemed to be thought of except the patients. Mrs. B. was in a fine stew packing her trunk. By dark we could see Newport Barracks burning, but could learn nothing of the men who defended it. You never did hear of such a night, I guess, as that was,—the citizen women screaming from every house, so loud that we could hear them, because their men were compelled to fight and, of course, to be killed without mercy; the terrified negroes constantly arriving; the thousand reports brought in each moment; the occasional firing of a gun by some very scared sentry; and always such a rushing to and fro.

I utterly refused to pack or budge unless the patients went too; but, at one o'clock, C. (hospital attendant) insisted on my sending my traps at least to the Fort, if I would not go myself. Flying men had begun to come in, some slightly wounded, all with alarming stories; and some of those at the fort which defends the town (Fort Heckman) could hear the Rebs chopping trees, etc.

So, I began to pack. War packing is a pretty hopeless job at any time; under such pressure it was impossible to choose. I wanted my treasures, and C. said to take the dry-goods; so, it was war between us. However, I managed to smuggle in my best traps; but I began to realise how inconvenient they are unless one is decidedly fond of them. We got through at last, and then went out to watch the beginning of the expected battle. There were not three hundred men in all, and the Rebs were said to be five thousand strong. The moon came up, and it was such a lovely scene,—the signals from the two forts and the gunboats (two at the station and one at Fort Macon), the frogs singing as if nothing were going on, and the air so warm and still. We sat for hours, and only when the morning broke went to bed. The patients had at last fallen asleep, and broad day light found them still sleeping. I had to give big doses of morphine to accomplish even that.

Well, the night was over, and the Rebels had not come, and everybody was quite worn out. The excitement was intense, cut off as we were from all communications, and just waiting to be "took." About ten in the morning news came that the Ninth Vermont and Mix's New Cavalry (I forgot to mention them) had crossed the Newport River, burned the railroad bridge, and come down on the other side to Beaufort. I must tell you first how this place lies: we are on a very narrow strip with Bogue Sound on one side and Calico Creek on the other; then another narrow strip, and then Newport River; so, you see they had a good distance to get round. They were soon brought over here, and people felt a little relieved to have some more help. At first it was supposed half of the men were killed or prisoners, but they have been gradually straggling back, so now but few, comparatively, are not accounted for,—only the Nineteenth Wisconsin has not been heard from. I'll bet they fought; that is a bully regiment, and we fear that all who were left are prisoners. Now here was another day and night,—constant alarms, everybody all ready for flight. Doctor gave shelter in one of the barracks to about a hundred negro women and children who had to be fed and cared for, besides the sick and tired soldiers pouring in all day; but at least we had more soldiers in the forts, though they were tired ones. Still the Rebels did not come. All day yesterday (Thursday) we could see fires in all directions, perhaps turpentine and perhaps homes of loyal men. About two we could see parties of people moving about on the opposite side of the creek a mile and a half away, and big fires too; now it seemed inevitable that we were to be "done took," and I guess no one lay down quite easy in his bed.

But morning found us all right, and, later, the *Spaulding* came with the Twenty-First Connecticut, old fighters, and, they say, good. Anyway, at two they, with the Ninth Vermont and Cavalry, started on an expedition; the cars took them up seven miles and left them to proceed to Newport Barracks on foot; of course, by this time the Rebels were miles away. I have no doubt reinforcements will be sent to our help from New Berne unless that is taken, and I reckon it is not, though it has been surrounded; but they have many forts and gunboats. All communication is cut off, the bridge burned and telegraph destroyed, so God knows how they may be; anyway, all are sure of a quiet night, and I have, as you see, a little leisure to tell you about it.

I have been so often reminded of Mrs. Bluebeard and her sister Ann, for there has been such a constant watching from high places for reinforcements, and my gallery has been the principal scene of action all the day: "Do you see any steamers?" "Nary a steamer,"—till the head was almost off. I believe Madam was going to have her head off; I've almost forgotten the *modus operandi*.

Through all this I have been so provoked that I could not get up one bit of a scare or even excitement; I could not even feel anxious. Of course, I could not sleep for the everlasting hubbub, but, I don't say it for boasting, I couldn't see it. It seemed to me quite a nice phase in war life. Had I really believed the Ninth and cavalry made a good stand and had really lost many men, I might have felt different; but as they once passed six months in Chicago as paroled prisoners, and Harper's Ferry was all the fight they ever were in, I believed they would skedaddle ingloriously, as I believe they did, and as we most of us here meant to. I may be unjust, but that is what I say. Anyway, one thing they did, and that was mean; they burned the long bridge behind them, completely cutting off the retreat of the cavalry and the Second Massachusetts (H. A.) and poor Wisconsin, so they had to swim for it; and it is said many of the Second boys were drowned; anyway, they are missing yet.

They talk of many wounded and killed, but they brought only three into Beaufort, and one or two have straggled in here. All that came I have in my ward. The Ninth had been recruited by four hundred; the recruits arrived at eleven and were attacked at twelve; rather soon to begin, but it is said they stood up well. It seems, though, that the most who are missing are the new ones. One sad story I have heard: two brothers stood side by side, and both were killed within a moment of each other; a hard sorrow for the poor parents at home. I fear I have not given you a very graphic account of what has really been quite an interesting episode in our life; but it is so hard to tell stories good. (For these skirmishes see *Official Records of the War of the Rebellion*, Series I. vol. xxxiii. p. 47.)

I sometimes am tempted to send you a nigger; I know such a nice servant, and she wants to go North. I have a little one to take care of my room and run my errands. If her nose were in order, she would be quite charming; but I am constantly charging on her for that, and it is quite wearing; especially, too, as I have to supply her the needful apparatus, which she is continually losing.

Morehead City, February 25 (1864).

I have had my hands full of wounded at last. I have twelve wounds today, all, I reckon, that were wounded in that *bloody* battle of Newport Barracks. My crowning was a Rebel who was brought to me today with a good Union ball through his lungs; such a gaunt, haggard, emaciated specimen of humanity you never have seen, because such kinds of men are never found up there; they are peculiar to North Carolina, a true type of all. When I should tell he was dirty, you could not then understand the word in its full sense; you must see a Southern soldier first to understand. I had him washed and cut and clothed, and now I hope to be able to approach him without having my nose tied up. The poor fellow, though, is very grateful and very sick. He was left, with another, when the Rebels retired at their leisure; but before they left him they stripped off all his clothes; they could not afford to leave even those. I have put him in a room with my pet patient, Will S., of the *gallant* Ninth. Now Willie is a real character, and I expect there will be some fun there; he has a ball in the back of his head. He makes so much fun of his wound and the way his face was pointed; often asks me if I had not rather be dressing that than his nose, which would probably have been the seat of the injury if he had minded his old mother and not run; but, he says, somehow the legs would go that way spite of all he could do. He declares that in the midst of it, thinking about her, he said to himself, "Land, she would run too, if she was here and saw all those darned Rebs after her;" and that was the last thought he had for some time. He is such a homely fellow, and with his shaved head and bandages would make a capital scarecrow. Poor man! it is doubtful if he gets well, and he knows his danger; but it doesn't stop his fun at all.

Another good patient I have is Tom G., of the same regiment. He is shot in the right arm, near the shoulder. There is constant danger of haemorrhage, and he is in intense pain (probably the nerve is severed); but he bears it splendidly, and is always ready to laugh. His companion is a cross Frenchman who had a bad wife and hates women; so, he kept his head always covered when I came near him and never spoke,—only moaned. He is slung up in an anterior splint and hates the "damned machine;" but somehow, lately, he has got to liking the "damned" women better, and really looks at me with smiles, and, today, asked me to write an English letter to his dear cousin Margy; so I think I have conquered him with kindness, and made him have a better opinion of women generally.

Morehead City, April 3 (1864).

All the boys want me to write their letters to you; but I tell them no, they must get some boy to write. I have to write for five of them every week, often several letters, and it is about as hateful a thing as they could set me at. When practice makes perfect, I shall be a good letter-writer before I die, if the war lasts awhile. I think, had I known this part of my duties, I never would have enlisted. Sergeant H. almost wore me out; he had so many kinsfolk, and every day somebody must be written to. It is so hard to express other people's thoughts. Smith's, now, are entertaining; he dictates and I write what he says, when I can for laughing."

The "terrible schoolma'ms" of the following letter do not appear in any earlier correspondence. Probably the letter referring to them has been lost.

Morehead City, May 6 (1864).

I have only a few moments just to tell you the Rebels have not got here yet, though some people are hourly expecting them; not so I. I still believe they will not venture here. The town is full of rumours and nothing is known. The train was cut off yesterday, and the wires severed; the last news was that they were fighting hard at New Berne, and that terrific Ram was there, and all sorts of horrid things.

For us, we are full of refugees; three hundred and fifty women and children came here the day after I last wrote you, and since then Bedlam has been let loose. The schoolma'ms seemed terrible, as I told you; but think of so many dirty women and children let into the grounds. They occupy two big barracks; some of them have not a change of clothes. They had only an hour's notice to quit Washington (N. C.). You cannot know anything of squalor till you see these people, all piping and chewing and crying everlastingly; perfectly satisfied to sit on the floor without making an effort to better their condition, only by an extra chew of snuff.

We can't even make them wash themselves or their clothes; everybody is busy doing for them, for something must be done. I never before knew anything of war horrors; you should see and hear them to believe. Some of these women's husbands have fallen into the Rebels hands; of course, they are murdered, as not a North Carolinian has escaped, they say. You have already seen how the Rebels treated the negroes; the men were marched out in squads, made to dig their own graves, and then murdered and thrown into them, one at a time. I saw a man yesterday who saw it. Every child, even, who was found with a bit of black on it was treated in the same way.

Our men at Plymouth were all stripped, and in an hour every Rebel was dressed in our uniform. Both Plymouth and Washington are destroyed, and, they say, Roanoke is also taken. All those places were won by such hard fighting and so hardly kept, so much life lost, and now to be given right up again! It is too bad; what do they mean to do?

I must tell you of my new charge. I have selected from the lot three of the lousiest, dirtiest, raggedest little things you ever saw in your life, and brought them here to take care of. The oldest, a girl, is blind, and so ignorant and forlorn. They had not a person in the world to take care of them, not a bed to sleep on; the little boys are really pretty, but such sights as they were when I brought them up here; not a spot on their bodies that isn't sore. Of course, the first thing I did was to strip them and burn everything they had on, and they were literally naked in the world. The mother and baby died a few days since, and the father is a soldier in the Second North Carolina, God knows where. I have been sewing my hand off to get something made for them, and now have them quite decent. I give them a scrub in soap and water every night, and the poor little things are looking more human now.

Of course, they are a great care; but I had to do it; those poor blind eyes were too strong for me. Her name is Angelico; she has a new coat and shoes for the first time, and is really smiling; but she has awfully dirty habits, and I tell you the "Heavenly Father feeling" comes in play often. I shall keep them till some provision can be made for them by the government, or the father can come for them. One of the soldiers will adopt the youngest if his father will give him up entirely."

The monotony of the summer's work was relieved, as occasion offered, by camping out on the ocean side of Shackelford Island (see earlier), where, with other women of the hospital staff, Mrs. von Olnhausen spent many a pleasant hour bathing, walking, and searching for shells and seaweeds.

August 22 (1864).

I have been to the sea for a day or two, and yesterday (Sunday) a big storm came; the tents are old and leaky and so Dr. Bellangee sent for us. The storm was fearful, and it is two miles to cross; but Dr. Cowgill thought it was safer in the boat than there, and such a sail as we had over! The sea was awful, and the wind, in gusts, dead ahead. Soon after we started I guess everyone wanted to be on shore again; but there was no going back without swamping, so on we came. We were two hours getting over and were wet to the pelt. Then the boat shipped water and had been at the wharf only a few moments when she sank, kerflop! I assure you I shall never go to sea in such a storm again.

I can't yet tell for certain about my coming home; though, unless pay day comes, it would be impossible anyway, for I would not go without a little money ahead. And I must tell you of a very foolish thing I did. That Mrs. C. (schoolma'm) who was here a while ago had a big wardrobe and no money; she came to me with such a pitiful story about her child, etc., and wanted me to buy some of her dresses. At first, I ridiculed the idea; but she was persistent and sorrowful; and finally, Mrs. B. also came and urged. I told her I was no judge of the worth anyhow; she said she would be umpire, and as she has kept store, etc., and is very shrewd, I thought she would be fair to me; so, I took three dresses and some laces.

Well, after I paid her and showed my bargain, everybody laughed at me; and I for once see the truth of "*a fool and her money.*" I guess nobody was ever so taken in! Wasn't it real shabby in Mrs. B., and she, too, laughs; and worse than all, C. told around among all the employees of the hospital that I was such a green woman; that I insisted on buying her clothes; she kept refusing, but it was no use, have them I would, and now she had to make fresh ones just to gratify my whims! So, all that pay went for nothing; as I certainly would never wear one of them here. You are real comforting in saying it's fortunate my children all died, when I mourned so for them! You can't know how I missed Franky; he was such a dear little boy. You ask what has become of all those people; they are scattered about in tents and shanties and live not half so good as pigs. I came across one woman yesterday, in my walk, who was living with her daughter and granddaughter under a quilt spread over a pole. It was just high enough to sit in, the bed was spread right in the sand, and such a bed! and such an unhappy old woman! as you may believe.

She was driven from a good home, where she had been born and expected to die. She had a nice farm, well stocked; but would be Union and so had to fly for her life. They robbed her of everything; but she says it doesn't matter much; she had rather be so than one of them! I have heard so many old women say the same thing; the young ones only seem bad! I have seen so much misery since I have been in North Carolina that I forget all I have ever seen before! Our Illinois farm was princely. It will either harden me to stone or else take away every bit of selfishness from me.

August 23 and September 4, 1864.
A fortnight ago I got so far along, and since then I'm hanged
if I've had a minute to write or do anything (only when I am
too tired) till today. The *nigs*, (in the laundry, of which she had
been put in charge), are more than I can stand; they bully me so
I don't know where I am. One of them told me this morning
"she'd give me a shakin down yet 'fore she got't rough"; which
sounds so respectful that I've been quite satisfied with myself
and my dignity ever since.

She is a miserable-looking little article, too, black as night, and
with such thick lips. I made her fold some dressing-gowns over
for the fifth time, and she thought that was once too often
considering she had washed them over twice! Now you can see
the good of giving me such a place. I'm no more fit to manage
them than those of their own colour. But this week has brought
me all right so far as work goes; I have made things shine, and
now defy anyone to find fault; they gave unconditional praise
on inspection this morning.

Morehead City, September 18, 1864.

This life is more monotonous now than I ever knew it before;
it's the same thing each day, varied a little, when the cars come,
with the hope of mail and the rumours of the fever which is
raging at New Berne. Some say it is the yellow fever and some
that it is congestive chills; anyway, it is alarming, as so far all
have died in a short time after being taken. I only half believe
the stories; but everyone who comes down seems tolerably
frightened, and many families are moving away. Thus far it is
confined mostly to citizens; few soldiers have been attacked. If
it should prevail to a great extent, of course it is my duty to go
there, and I suppose I shall. I have no fear of it, and only doubt
whether I could do much good; but still I shall try.

September 24, 1864.
I must write you a short letter, fearing you will be anxious
about the fever at New Berne; so far, we are all well here. One
woman who came from New Berne with the disease has died,
and one case has appeared in the hospital; but still it seems almost impossible that it can prevail here, this is such a healthful

place and so clean too, thanks to Dr. Bellangee. He stayed here only one day, and then was ordered up to New Berne to take charge of the Health Department. He is made President of the board and is doing sweeping work there; he wrote today that he is making a fearful amount of enemies, and is constantly exposed to danger, but he would shirk nothing; that he considered it his duty as long as God spared him.

He wrote to his wife and me together, begging me to stay by through this crisis; that he should feel such courage if he knew I was here to do my share. He would not hear of my going to New Berne. You see I had my papers all arranged to go Monday on the *Petrel*, that sails from this port; but I found him so sad about it I gave it up. I had anticipated so much pleasure in being at home; but that must be deferred now till another time. I hope the fever will soon abate, and then I shall think again of starting. I will send a bulletin every few days, so don't be worried about me.

September 28, 1864.

I am sure you will be glad to hear from me if only a few words. I am so sorry to tell you that our dear doctor was brought back here yesterday so sick that I can't tell you how he is. That fearful fever, no one can say how it will terminate; but his symptoms are not so bad as some who have come here.

September 30, 1864.

I did not write yesterday, as it was such an anxious day with us all. Doctor was very sick all day, and I could not leave him for a moment. Today he is still bad; but the symptoms are all encouraging, and if he holds out as he is now till after four o'clock this afternoon, we feel as if all danger would be passed,—I mean the frightful part; of course he will be fearfully prostrated, and it will require all his iron constitution to carry him through till Monday, when he will begin to rally.

Till you are with it you can have no idea of this dreadful fever; nothing else approaches it except cholera. The effect upon the spirits would alone be distressing enough; but then the agony of the patient, and his consciousness of the danger add so much to the horror. No one expects to live, and when the black vomit comes that look of despair with the "There is no show for me any longer" makes your heart just full.

The news from New Berne is bad enough today; the fever seems on the increase and the weather is still warm; this morning was fearful. We are still spared here; no cases except those brought from there; and though the doctor so far is the only hopeful one, yet there were many more cases in New Berne cured this week than last. Perhaps they treat it better; though it is often the fact in this epidemic that after the third week the proportion of cures is much greater. It seems it appeared as early as the first of September, but they have been trying to keep it dark; called it congestive chills, etc., and took no steps to remove the causes even, till Dr. Bellangee went there.

The world has to thank Dr. ———, a Massachusetts man, who has been Health Officer there, for all this. He has allowed everything to accumulate and has never remonstrated,—not even with the Quartermaster, who filled in a whole square of the dock with condemned beef, pork, and vegetables. The barrels were thrown in just as they were, full, and were then covered with about three feet of earth. The fever originated there, and not one in that quarter got well. It then spread all over the town. Moreover, the town has never been drained, and every vault and sink, even of the hospital, is in an awful condition.

It's too bad that so many lives should be sacrificed to such wanton neglect. It is said that dead hogs and dogs and other animals come floating down those two sluggish streams that surround New Berne (the Neuse and Trent) and make into an eddy at the piers; there they lie, putrid, till they finally melt away. What can one hope from such a town? I would gladly go there and do my share of it. Can I be too glad, though, that I am here to nurse the doctor? He needs me so much. The boys turn pale when I speak of going; so, unless something particular happens, I shall not go at present.

Isn't it singular that black people do not take the fever? Some yellow ones have had it; but not one black. The poor refugees die with it on short notice. Those all-suffering people have had more than their share,—measles, small-pox, worms, and now fever; not many will be left to tell the tale of suffering by the time winter is over.

What can the poor things do, so broken now, in their crowded tents,—God help them!

October 2, 1864.

What do you think the New Berne paper of yesterday says?

> Some people for some reason are trying to get up a pan-
> ic, saying we have some infectious disease here, which is
> perfectly false; typhoid and swamp fevers are prevalent,
> but to no alarming extent, and there is no epidemic pre-
> vailing.

Is it not a shame to publish such lies? Friday and yesterday each
there were twenty-five burials, all of yellow fever. Whole families are found dead in their houses; four were found yesterday,
the wife lying across the feet of her dead husband, and both
children dead beside them; and with this knowledge, to say
such lies! I hope to come home this fall, but that will depend
on how long this sickness lasts. When the fighting commences
at Wilmington, I suppose I can't come; and, if it is late, the long
sail in these vile tempests is rather an objection.

Morehead City, October 5, 1864.

The news from New Berne grows worse each day, and sick
men are continually being brought here; but I have not time
to look after those in my ward now; Dr. Bellangee claims me
first and all.

Dr. Hand wrote yesterday:

> The fever grows worse; God only can help us. I'm dread-
> fully blue and exhausted, I can scarcely get upstairs to
> bed after my work is done.

He is medical director of this department, and so far, the only
surgeon who has escaped; but they say he is worn to a skeleton.
After Friday, this port is closed to all except gunboats. There is
no doubt that Wilmington is to be attacked; so now God only
knows when I shall get home. The quarantine is twenty days,
even for letters, in New York; so I fear you will be very anxious
about me.

Morehead City, October 14, 1864.

I don't know how I can tell you the mournful news of our dear
friend's (Dr. Bellangee s) death. My last letter was hopeful of his
recovery; but an hour after it had gone he was taken worse and
suffered more than I am sure any poor mortal deserved. I can
hardly remember the particulars now, it was so pitiful to us all.

He suffered constantly, notwithstanding quantities of chloroform, till three in the morning, when he died; his screams will never be forgotten.

Last night another very sick patient was brought to me,—a Mrs. N., mother of Mrs. Colonel A. of Boston. The colonel and she have both died this week, and no one would take in or keep this poor old woman, who has the fever; so, Doctor (Palmer) and I concluded we must. I dread another such trial, of course; but what can one do when all are suffering so? I also have a sick doctor from New Berne Hospital, so I can only keep on working until God sends us frost.

Our hospital is full of sick, though so far only those are taken who have been brought from New Berne; no case has originated here. In Beaufort, it is different; there the fever appeared of itself, the first victims being Colonel A. and his wife. I have had, besides all this nursing, to pack everything for Mrs. Bellangee, think for her, and take charge of the House; and now I am at the station with her waiting for the ship to sail that will take her from this sorrowful place. She is so disappointed that I will not go North with her; but I see clearly my duty is here. I could not leave Dr. Palmer now in his trial.

This is the first time I have sat down today, and with no sleep last night I feel drowsy and stupid enough; but I would not let the ship sail without these few words. I know you think of me often now; but don't feel anxious. I am perfectly well with the exception of being tired, and am really glad to be where I can make comfort to so many. I can't tell you how grateful I felt when the rumour went out that I, too, was to leave today. The boys all came to me with: "Mrs. O., don't leave us, you are all we have now; what can we do without you?" and their gladness when I told them I would stay! Dr. Palmer just kissed my hands and went away. I am real egotistical, I know; but I can't help it; I am a little weaker than usual from being overtired."

This "little weakness" developed quickly into yellow fever, of which she had an extremely serious case. When sufficiently convalescent to bear the journey, she was taken North to the frosts and healing air of Lexington.

Chapter 7

Returning to Morehead City in December, 1864, Mrs. von Ol-nhausen remained there until early in the following April, when she was transferred, first to Beaufort and afterwards to Smithville, North Carolina. During this period the war came to an end through the surrender of Lee, and President Lincoln was assassinated. The demoralization inseparable from the ending of a great war made itself plainly felt in the hospitals; and the disorganisation of these last months was almost as great as that of her first experience, at Alexandria. Remaining with the hospital at Smithville as long as there was any need for her services, she at last received her discharge in the closing days of August, 1865. Laden with birds, animals, curios, and kindred "traps," and accompanied by a "Contraband" man-servant, she returned in the late summer to the welcome of her Lexington homes.

Morehead City, Sunday, December 11, 1864.
Back once more in my own room, so much bluer than I expected to be. I half determined not to write at all, I felt so homesick. I arrived here yesterday morning, after being a whole week on my journey, thoroughly tired, for it was such a roundabout way to come. Most of the time we had bad weather and not a soul for company; so, it made the time seem even longer.
I left New York Monday, and had the usual tiresome ride to Baltimore; but the cars were detained, so the boat had already left for Fortress Monroe, and I must wait till the next day. I went to Barnum's, and the first stupid thing I did was when the clerk asked me my name. I could not, for a moment, remember it at all; he stared suspiciously at me, till at last I told him. I also said I wanted the valise and largest trunk sent to my room. When they were brought up I found the trunk had been opened, and the blankets taken off. I asked why, and the porter said it was

too hard to carry with them on; but afterwards, when I came to open the trunk, I found the reason. I suppose, from my hesitation and having so much luggage, they took me for a "torpedo woman" or some kind of a fire-critter; and I did not blame them, I was so stupid.

I had a nice walk round town next day, and at four we left. The boat was crowded and my berth was right over the engine, so it was pretty warm; but a shower came in the night and gave me a wetting, through the skylight, which cooled me off. We arrived about seven in the morning at the fortress, and found there were no outside boats for two or three days; so, I took the canal. It rained so I could not go about at all, excepting to the provost's and quartermaster's; and at ten we left for Norfolk. In two hours, we were there and had to fly round to get transportation, as the boat was ready to start. It still rained, and I was by this time pretty uncomfortable, as you may believe. In fact, I never before started from home so badly prepared for a journey; I had nothing comfortable. You know I had no change of anything. The boat was a dirty little affair, and I was so glad I had enough of my own to eat.

That night we got nearly to the mouth of the canal, where we found a gunboat sunk, and a big boat jammed with her in attempting to pass. It was fast, and the prospect was rather dismal, as her own machinery was powerless, owing to the wheels being fast, and our boat seemed too small to move her; but they put on steam, bumped at her for two hours, and at last crowded her out. Then we changed boats, as there was no room to turn. She still had to poke the big boat out of the canal, so it was nearly morning before we started again.

Dr. Palmer's Lieutenant-Colonel Clark was on board; he had just been on a raid into Rebeldom, had captured all the forces he met, together with ninety bales of cotton, eight wagons, twenty mules (he had to shoot those, for he had no room to bring them back); had burned a great quantity of stores, and had pitched a hundred sacks of salt into the river. He had to work in a hurry, for there was a large force in reserve, and every moment he was expecting them. His force was very small,— only two or three hundred in all; and just as they were off the Rebels came in sight. He was most proud of his success, and well he might be; everyone here praises him.

When we reached Roanoke, we found everybody in great excitement there. All the soldiers had been taken away, and most of the gunboats; also, the regular boat to New Berne. So again, we had to wait till two that night before the mail-boat came down to take us. I wandered about the island alone, and poked into many shebangs. One woman was just eating dinner, and invited me to partake. I was cold and hungry after the walk; and although the tablecloth was a salt sack, and dirty at that, and the fork had but one prong, and she had only corn bread and *biled* pork and greens, I laid aside fastidiousness and sat with her. The coffee really did taste good, though the sugar looked dubious and there was no milk.

But it was wet and warm, washed the grub down, and made the old lady happy, because I was a Northerner and not proud. She was very strong Union, had suffered all that one can, was seventy-four years old, and had not one cent left in the world. Her clothes she buried before she left, and was next day going back to Plymouth to try to find them. She was very well known there, and liked; and when the town was being taken two officers, knowing her, and how much she would suffer if left, took her and ran down to the boat, she being the last to escape. One of the officers was captured. The run nearly killed the old lady, she said. With the fright and hurry, her breath was clean gone, and she fell down helpless. She "likes us Yanks enough."

It was a real cold day, but I kept walking; it was better than staying in the lonely boat with nobody but two "Chinary" girls to stare at one. I went back at sundown, and the old lady was so anxious for fear I should miss the way (as if one could in that little, one-horse town) that she went to the boat with me. I was sorry, afterwards, that I did not take her on board and give her some clothes; she would have been so glad. I gave her some money and she was very grateful.

The Sound was rough, and everybody was sick, and there were no berths on board. The benches, of course, were as hard as boards could make them. In fact, the last bed I slept on till I got here was at Baltimore. The night before I passed on the narrowest kind of a seat, all "booted and spurr'd," and the consciousness of a tumble never left me.

Morehead City, December 25 (1864).
I should feel "meaner than pusley" for not having written if

I had not a tip-top excuse. I never did accomplish so much, I think, in one week before. Tuesday brought your letter, also the box; but then I was too deep in Christmas preparations to think of anything else. You know we have never been paid yet. The black women were perfectly destitute, they really had nothing to wear,—and such unmitigated growling. So, Doctor said I had better take some bed-ticks and give them dresses; also, some coarse underclothing. The Sanitary, furthermore, had given me, a long time ago, some bed-sacks of lapping. I knew it was no use to give them anything unmade, as they would botch it so; so, I commenced and, more than that, executed the gigantic undertaking of making the clothing all up. Now that was a work. I sewed literally night and day. Friday, I was in despair, and made a sewing-bee; called all the neighbours in, and so by night got nearly done.

Besides working for the *nigs*, I had all those refugee things to fix up and arrange. It took some judgment to parcel them out; but everything was done by last night. Moreover, the box came yesterday, just in time to distribute.

Our harbour has been full of the fleet. It was splendid: sixty ships and eight monitors. They sailed out Friday and Saturday week for Wilmington. Doctor took us down to see them, and we went on board the double-turreted monitor, the *Monadnock*. How I wish you could have seen it! I don't see how anything could hurt her;—four feet of wood, and seven inches of wrought iron, and such turrets, and such guns! The shells were fifteen inches and they carried five miles, sure. Well, they all sailed out and we expected, Sunday, to hear the attack, for though it's ninety miles we can hear them; but no guns came.

Tuesday the transports, with General Butler's whole force, commenced coming in for coal and water; they had been lying off Wilmington sixteen days, on half rations, expecting the fleet. Of course, there was somebody wrong, as usual. The men were suffering terribly, crowded into the ships, expecting to be only five days and not allowed to bring even a change of clothes, not a knapsack even; all was to be sent after them. They had waited, as I say, sixteen days, and many were sick. Then we had an awful storm and the coldest weather I've ever known here; so many of them were frostbitten. The ships were brought to the wharf, one by one, and the men allowed to land while the ships were cleaned. They were like wild men, and no one could blame them. Our hospital was full of them, wanting everything,—officers and men alike; for the little that was to be bought in these stores was sold at once.

The day of my "bee" I was sitting here with a room full of women, when who should come in but Dr. Barnes (medical inspector of the whole troops here); I was so glad to see him, and he seemed pleased, too. He stayed to tea, and was too glad to get something to eat; for they had had nothing but salt pork and hard tack for many days. He said it was the first "square" meal he'd eaten for a long while. He appealed to the benevolent ladies of Lexington, said he remembered them, and claimed their charity; for he was both lousy and dirty, and did not even blush to own it. He left that for General Butler to do, who got them into that condition. I had nothing for him but a clean handkerchief; but Dr. Palmer gave me a suit of "Sanitary" for him, and he went away rejoicing.

They sailed yesterday afternoon, so are now fighting. We hear the guns all day very plainly; the firing is continuous. The news has come that Fort Fisher has surrendered, and the troops are landing. I suppose by this you will have heard of the trick played on them of the ship being chased, rigged like an English vessel, loaded with powder. Friday night it was accomplished; we felt and heard the report here; it must have been terrible there. Everyone started from sleep; the report is that it shattered the town awfully. (As a matter of fact, it was a complete failure.) We are all so anxious here to know the result of today's fighting. It would be a nice Christmas gift to the Nation when we could gain that Secesh place. (The Union forces were repelled at Fort Fisher on December 25, 1864, but took the fort by assault on January 15, 1865.)

Monday (December 26).

I was stopped yesterday, for Kitty P. came for me to go sailing; and then in the evening we went to the negro meeting, where we laughed our fill. How I wish you could go to a real *nig* meeting and hear them exhort. One man kept asking if we did not hear the "strumpets of de Lord a-calling and a-calling: 'I hears the strumpets all round me, Bress de Lord forever.'" Then he "prayed de Lord to fire up his coal;" I guess he is a fireman. Today I'm having a grand row with the *nigs*. They got so stupid and behind hand I've sent two off, and the work drags.

Morehead City, January, 1865.
They say the paymaster comes tomorrow, and will pay us four months if we will sign four months rolls; but all declare they won't. It will soon now be twelve months' pay due us. Isn't it real mean? It is so in no other department. Some of the men have such pitiful letters from their families, wanting everything and blaming them, saying that other women must get their money. I see a good many swollen faces after the mail comes in; and some of the letters make me cry, too. There is certainly money somewhere. Some lay it to the paymaster, who is speculating in the coupons, and some charge poor Butler with the whole sin.

Morehead City, Thursday, January (?19), 1865.
Happy! Two hundred wounded and I the only wound-dresser in the ward; they are just arriving. I shall have all I can do now, and the best kind, too! Send me a box of all you know I want for wounded men, especially rags and long bandages.

Morehead City, Sunday, January (?29), 1865.
I have forty-four beds. I have taken the ward just back of the carriage house, Ward 6. It is right clean, one of the best of the lot, and I have such good attendants and have everything about my own way. Dr. Palmer has much more faith in me, of course, than I deserve; but I can't help seeing myself that there never was a ward of badly wounded men doing so well as these; he can't say enough about it. I am sure of one thing, that I have lost nothing in being down here; my judgment is clearer, and my nerves are steadier than ever.
How I wished today after I was ready for inspection that you could have looked in and seen us all,—the men so jolly and clean and comfortable. They look to me for everything. Doctor has so much to attend to that he really leaves more to me than he ought; so, they think I'm supreme. Sometimes he doesn't come in all day, unless I send for him.
How you would like one old Englishman I have; his arm is amputated at the elbow, and such a job never was done before. It is meant for a flap, and I guess they took the whole meat down to the hand and just rolled it up and sewed it there. He is so enthusiastic about the battle. It was a splendid charge, taking that

fort (Fisher); the men were glorious. He was not wounded until just as they were entering; he had just got upon the parapet. His captain ran up to him; he said: "Never mind, Captain, this is worth an arm, we've beat 'em. If we had gone back as we did before, I would have wished it was my life. I'll pull through it;" and he has, sure enough. One of my men has been wounded in six different battles; such a banged-up fellow you never saw. Now he has a bullet through the wrist and one through the side; he is very sick, but is so brave about it. I like to take care of such men.

At first, I had some Rebels in my ward; but I made the doctor take them out and fill the ward up with Union. The Rebels make me so mad, and are so presuming, too. It was always "Madam, will you look at my wound?" Now I didn't want to see their wounds, unless they were going to die from them. You can't tell how wicked that book, (there is no other reference to show what "book" is meant), has made me toward them. I can't be good, and it makes me furious to see them treated just as well as our men. The only way I could spite them was to give them one less blanket than ours had.

One little boy I keep; he declared before all the Rebels that he and all his family were always Union, that he never wanted to fight, was a conscript and was glad to get away from them. He said: "I know if they get me again I shall catch it for saying this, but I'll never go back to them, I'd rather die here." When we were having the others moved, he begged me not to send him with them. "I shall die sure if I leave you, Mrs. Woe" (that is a hard name).

But my most interesting patient is a man who has had resection of the larger bone of the left arm. He is such a splendid fellow. He has the rheumatism in both legs, so he can't move them, and ought to be cross as a bear; but instead of that just looks like a saint. He is married, and I have to write his letters, and he dictates so lovelily. By the way, there never was a prettier room than mine. It is too lovely (I mean for down here). My decorations are so jolly, and my dog barks all night, and altogether I have a nice life, and if we only could have warm weather my cup would be quite full.

I must tell you about the war between our two chaplains. It is too funny. B., the old man, is a presidential chaplain, he says; the other, L., is some side branch. I don't understand how he comes in; but they are so jealous of each other. First one orders the house closed when the other is going to preach, and then the other retaliates; so, between them we get no preaching. Last Sunday night B. ordered the fire and the lights put out. L. pitched into him and then complained to Dr. Palmer. Old man denied his guilt; so, Dr. Palmer ordered them both before him at eleven next day. Each refused to meet the other; but Doctor told them unless they obeyed he would order them under arrest.

So, they came, sword in hand. Doctor could not get in even a side cut. At last he got the floor for a moment, and then he told them he never had too much faith in Christian doings, etc., but now what little he had was destroyed. "He was about sick now of any chaplain, and unless they stopped immediately he would report them both at Washington. It was a disgrace, etc." He ran them hard for an hour, until both promised to do better in future.

Next day a man was to be buried. B. waited at the office gate to join the escort, instead of going to the dead house. L. got the start of him, was on the spot, and came along booted and spurred. B. flew out, ordered him off, etc. L., having the fear of the law, meekly, but with black looks, dismounted and proceeded, with the help of another man, to boost old B. on; then the stirrups were too long, so they must be fixed. All this time the dead man and escort were waiting. Finally, when all was adjusted, the *cortège* started; and then B. found riding was not so easy as it looked, and wobbled about in the saddle till he nearly rolled off. One of the bearers came to his help, led the beast, and held the rider stiff. So, at last the procession passed out of sight. I thought we must die laughing. B. was "poorly" and quite lame for two or three days after that ride.

Yesterday L.'s removal came, so B. is bigger than a gobbler today, talks about his stupendous duties, etc.; but when the bugle sounded for church the poor old thing's ears didn't do their duty, and his watch had been forgotten to be wound; so, when the people had sat for half an hour, they went home. When nearly an hour had passed, he scrambled off himself to church and found it empty; he waited another hour before he knew he was too late. This was a poor beginning to his "stupendous duties."

I cannot mention anything in the box that I do not particularly want, especially the eatables (which you will believe). I wish you could have looked in and seen us after we had dragged out the last parcel and were resting from our work. We all sat on the floor and commenced eating. Doctor *would* taste of everything, and how we did eat! We had to open just a bottle of that currant wine; it was so good, and we felt pretty tired, if we were *not* sick. After all, we could not decide which cake was best, or whether the cake was better than the cheese, or the pie best of all; and you will no doubt be disgusted to know that we ate a whole one between us.

Monday evening, I gave a little feast in my room, had the Palmers and some others, and myself. I made chocolate, and Mrs. Palmer made some hot biscuits. You can't know how they tasted with the butter; everyone agreed in declaring they never tasted anything like them. C. had two chickens roasted and shot six robins. I never saw people enjoy a supper so much; one must live down here and as we do to know that. We had the supper in C.'s room; he took out his bed, and the table looked splendid. We had celery, too; and the pies and cake and olives and cheese and pickles couldn't be beat,—but, oh, that bread and butter! After supper, we played euchre and whist till quite late; so you see it was a real Northern affair, and ought to have been noticed in the papers.

My refugee treasures are priceless. I am packing such a nice box to send down to the light-house; everything pretty I've reserved for my little Caledonia Royal, the keeper's youngest daughter, and the little half-witted girl, Mary Francis G. I've sent Mary Francis warm clothes and some of the playthings. I sent the ball to her little brother. He is a nice little boy, about three, but smokes all the time. Mrs. G. says it costs her more than a dollar a week to keep her and the children in tobacco. Send on your missionaries!

My ward is really doing splendidly. I have lost only one man, and that was inevitable; nothing could have saved him; his whole spine was affected by a grape shot. All the amputations are nearly healed. These barracks are so good on account of ventilation. They have been rather cold, but I guess our worst cold is over, and there is no more smell of wounds than if I had none, though there are forty-four, and almost all bad cases. We have had any quantity of inspectors, directors, etc.; all are so pleased with our hospital.

Orders have come today to extend its capacity to six hundred, immediately, by tents; so, tomorrow they will commence putting them up. This looks like work in North Carolina; and the constant arrival of troops makes it so animated here. Twelve hundred of the Constructing Corps arrived Sunday, and are camped close to us,—pontoons, and mules (400) that roar all the time. We have to keep a guard all around the grounds to prevent the rascals from stealing everything. I expect to have all the work I want; for the care of the wash-room is no light duty, with so many clothes to look after. I expect never to have a minute when we get full.

February 9, 1865.

C. and Doctor have been off the past two days, trying to find a place to pitch our tents, as it is decreed that we are really to leave here and tent it somewhere. They have about decided on a place a mile out of Beaufort. How I do hate it! Had it been the beach (on Shackelford Island, where the summer camp had been), I'd have been satisfied, though the impossibility of transportation made that useless to think of; but Beaufort is such a fleay, dirty-smelling hole, and full of Secesh and rum-holes, and gambling of all kinds going on there, the whole thing will become demoralised like that Beaufort hospital. Doctor looks anxious, and I am worn enough. As we lived last summer with every convenience, tent life was jolly. We were perfectly isolated and so independent; but it is another matter to live in a crowd, as we shall there; it is like living on the housetops.

The outrage of turning us out seems greater every day, and the spite of it is too much. To think that today a surgeon of a *nig* regiment has come in and taken one of our barracks (mine that I moved my wounded men from) and filled it up with his sick men; and yet they say they must have them for military purposes, when we could have and should have taken the same men if we had stayed. I can't see the difference or the justice.

I had a letter from one of my wounded men at New Berne, and he put on the direction "not to be pronounced like the numeral, but literally *o n e*." It seems they have to dress each other's wounds now. You will be glad that they had not to sleep on the ground, as we first heard; the sick really did, but this academy is a wounded ward and kept alone for that, and they had no wounds, so it was fortunately empty.

Perhaps you will be glad to know, too, that Dr. Hand, medical director, sent me word by Dr. Palmer that his nine surgeons, after examining those wounds, said they had never seen wounds so well dressed and such bad wounds so soon getting well; and, for himself, that I was the best wound-dresser in the country. I feel uncommonly satisfied, as these men a year ago were all opposed to female nurses and "poohed" at the idea of one being useful. It is rumoured today that Longstreet is at Goldsboro' with fifteen thousand men; if so, we must soon have more wounded, as twenty thousand have left New Berne these last few days. They have not even a provost-guard left there; all are taken to the front.

How I shall mourn for my dear little room; it looks so friendly tonight. You'd die with the traps, but they are such treasures to me, and each has its story. My owl looks down with approving eyes as I write. My crow almost caws, and my furniture is all so jolly, if it is pine boards covered with an old dress.

Morehead City, February 18 (1865).
I want to tell you of the arrival of the box, which came last night, much to my joy and the comfort of my patients. Rags had become so scarce I was picking up the bits blowing about the land. I never was in such straits before. The Sanitary Department had not even one of their old bandages to spare me. No delicacies ever looked so good to me as those rags.

We are terribly excited here just now; they threaten to break up the hospital and turn us all over to Beaufort. How mad we shall be to go to those dirty traps; but Sherman's commissary general is here, this is to be the supply base, he has already taken possession of most all the private buildings outside the grounds, and now wants these. Won't it be too bad to have such desecration? However, I've hopes it will take more than the General of New Berne to do it.

My wounded men are doing splendidly. So far, we have lost only one, which is surprising, for I never saw worse wounds; but I guess it did us all good not to have any wounds for so long; we take all the better care of them now. A good many Rebs have died, for they are in bad condition every way; and then I never have done any of them, except the two in my ward,—the little boy without the arm and the carotid-artery man. These two everybody said must die, so I thought I'd make them live.

It's the little one who calls me Mrs. Woe; the old Englishman calls me Mrs. Hoe; the man without the foot, Roe; and the man with the arm, Mrs. No; as to all the other names, I can't tell them; everything which has an O in it seems to fit. They are a grateful set of boys as ever lived, and I feel never tired of doing for them. In fact, we all have to spring night and day almost; we never had so much before. I wish I could get rid of the old laundry; but the fear of some disagreeable old cat makes me rather do it myself. I mean someday, though, to take a little walk; it's long now since I've been out of the gate.

Morehead City, March 1 (1865).
I did not write Sunday, and, how could I? Such discouraging news as we got that day. I just could do nothing after Doctor came and said our hospital was to be broken up. Is it not too bad? Every day since, the news has been fluctuating: now it is to be broken up altogether, now transferred to Beaufort,—to New Berne,—and the last news today is that it is to be transferred bodily to Smithville (or field), opposite Fort Fisher, on the seashore. Now this may all, or part, or none, be true; but still we are in an exercised state of mind, to say the least. We were just all so satisfied and don't want any change, and everything is going on so well. I never in all my hospital life was so nearly happy; everything and everybody is just right.

I suppose you are tired to death of my wounded, but how can I ever tire of them? I never saw such wonderful results before. We have not lost a man, though we had such terrible cases; and when I look around and see them all so cheerful and grateful, I am glad I am strong enough to be an army nurse. I expect you will think I am the greatest egotist in the world; but how can I help being a little exultant?

We have all sorts of visitors.—Dear me, one more telegram has just come that we are to move at once, tomorrow morning; everything must be moved, everything packed, the commissary takes possession at once. We are ordered to New Berne. How I do hate it, there of all places; I can't tell you how I feel. What disposition they will make of me I don't know; if possible, I shall stick to Doctor.

Morehead City, March 5 (1865).

The final telegram came, and we were to leave for New Berne Thursday morning at eight o'clock; cars were to be punctual, and every patient must be at once transferred to Foster Hospital. I was up at four o'clock; and by eight had every ward dressed and ready, and those who were to be removed on beds made comfortable for the journey. I rushed to my room, not even waiting for my breakfast, to make myself ready to accompany them; for I was to go and remain overnight, at least, to see that they were made comfortable. All the while the packing was going on,—all beds were returned to the store-room; all linen sent to the wash-room; all medicines packed and stored: such were the orders. It was confusion of the worst sort, such hurrying about, such anxious waiting.

So, we waited and waited till four; when a telegram came that the patients were not to be sent till the next morning. Now see again the confusion! The medical director arrived, beds were again unpacked, fresh linen issued, supper prepared, and, although no one wanted to leave, wretchedness and tiredness were on every face. You know how hard it is to wait. Some that had not been out of bed before, excepting long enough to have it made, had been all day sitting up and were fairly sick by the time I could get them in bed. That evening, Dr. M., the medical director, said he thought, after all, the worst sick and all the wounded would, for a time at least, be left; so, I went right down and told the men; you can't know how glad they were.

Next morning, I went in to dress them, when Dr. Palmer came and asked me how many it would be safe to take. I told him of Dr. M.'s promise; he said they had another telegram ordering all that could travel to come at once. He took all but twelve with him; so short a notice that I had not time to dress half their wounds. Then, when packed in the cars, they lay there four hours without dinner before they were finally taken to New Berne. Again, the ward was all torn up, as that one, being more isolated, was wanted for the quartermasters; so, I took Division

2, and worked all day to get it in order; still Doctor made me hold on.

Yesterday (Saturday) I had everything ready, but a big rain came up; and today it is too cold to move them; so they still lie in the old, dismantled ward.

Meantime I am more than discouraged; I am utterly disgusted with the selfishness of these men. Was ever such an outrage on our soldiers? The wards that have been emptied of our poor sick and wounded fellows were immediately filled with the dirtiest niggers you ever laid eyes on,—not even employees of the army, but hangers-on and followers from the Tennessee and Sherman's army; such dirt and filth cannot be equalled. The third ward is filled with ox-bows, tent poles, and wagon tyres,—hundreds of old traps. Not a white man or even a black soldier brought in; the whole is for spite. The quartermasters and commissary saw with envious eyes the front row of buildings, all houses built before the war, and claimed them as quarters for themselves.

Of course, the doctor refused; then they set to work to take everything, wrote to General Schofield that they were all needed for military purposes, and wanted his order at once. He, knowing nothing of the truth, sent it, and now we have been staving them off just to get time till he comes, which he was expected to do today to see for himself and decide for us. Meantime, when the hundred and fifty who were sent from here arrived in New Berne, four hundred men had already arrived from different regiments, and only provision made for our lot; they coming last, the most of them had to lie round in churches and anywhere they could settle, most of them without even blankets. If this is justice, I hate it forevermore.

Dr. Palmer went to New Berne last night to return today; but instead of him comes a telegram to be ready to store seventy hospital tents. Now, whether this means breaking up here or extending this one, we can none of us guess till he comes back in the morning. Such a state of uncertainty as we are in is decidedly unpleasant.

The town is full of troops, and the hubbub outside is worse than in. These officers keep coming to the houses and saying, "When will this be vacated?" so arrogantly. They stand before our doors and say what they intend to do when they get the quarters. If they are remonstrated with, they fall back on "We're from Sherman's army," as if that could cover all enormities. I am getting about sick of Sherman's army, if this is the way we are to be treated by them.

My men are all ill today; the news from their comrades and expectation of being served in the same way are enough to make them so. One of them died last night; we had never thought of his dying from his wound, but the excitement of Thursday and thinking he had got to leave his doctor and nurse were too much for him. They all cried so much that morning, and two men who were taken away on stretchers went weeping like children; think now what a trial for me, and of my anxiety about them! Two more I have very little hope of; they have both failed so these two days, and my carotid-artery man, that I was so bound should live, grows worse every hour.

I was in hopes he would live, though he was a Rebel, for Doctor's sake; and I am sure he would, except for this; but he was foolish enough to believe that no one could save him but me, and he cries about all the time. He doesn't give his old answer to my morning greeting, "I'm right piert, madam" any longer; just his lips tremble, and he says, "I'm bad off, I am losing courage." I hate to be in the ward now, but still I do my best to cheer them up."

In the interval between this and the following letter the transfer from Morehead to Beaufort evidently was made.

Beaufort, N. C., April 9, 1865.

As I am going to write a real growling note, I, of course, don't expect it to be read except in private circles; but this has been such a real Pandemonium this first week that I must "speak in meeting." I told you last Sunday that our dear doctor (Palmer) had left for Goldsboro' for an indefinite time, leaving us in charge of a drunken, ignorant, bad man without a particle of principle or judgment. Well, to begin with, Monday he did not rise till twelve o'clock; not another surgeon on the grounds and so many sick patients. I felt equal to the wounds; but still, as I had two cases of haemorrhage, it would be rather satisfactory to have a surgeon one could speak to.

Well, I never had a surgeon in my ward of fifty patients till Thursday, when Dr. Salter, post-surgeon,—and such a good man,—came to the rescue. I met him and told him how it was; as he is a great friend of Dr. Palmer s, he quickly volunteered to tend the wounded for a few days. He was needed by that time, as I'd given all the medicine I had in the ward, and, of course, could not make a prescription. So far, good. In the meantime, C. (attendant) has been very sick, not so bad as last spring, but sick enough to need constant care. He pulled through without a doctor; I knew what to do for him.

I told you a telegram had come that we were to take five hundred patients; they never got here till tonight; God help the poor souls now. They came cold and hungry. C. went to the doctor and said, "These men must have something to eat when they land, they have been short of rations all this time;" and he answered, "Damn it, a man can live a week without eating." But C. did, for all that, have a good hot supper for them. Only a hundred have landed; the wind blows so they could not get them on the lighters. The boat lies in the stream two miles off. But this is not the worst; there are a hundred and fifty without a bed or blanket to sleep on, and, what is more, no prospect of one. You see what they have to expect,—those other four hundred who have been lying seasick and heart sick and hungry on the swash for two or three days. Isn't it damnable? The churches were ordered to be taken for them, but no other provision has been made.

Whether it is the fault of medical purveyor or director I can't say; but certain it is there is no one here to make an effort. You can't know our loss in Dr. Palmer; had he been here, all would have been right. There are seventy tents pitched with only the sand to lie on. If we had one blanket apiece, it might do; but we have not one. I have cried and stormed and raved till now I have come to my room and won't even hear a sound. I say, God help them; and the drunken wretch has throughout behaved like an imbecile. I hope he will get his reward when the war is over.

Positively this week has been worse than any Alexandria doings. I could not begin to tell you all the annoyances, but will give one little item: though we had so good cause for rejoicing (over Lee's surrender), still, with so many sick men, it was no time to illuminate the hospital, especially this one, which in case of fire has only one narrow stairway, and has, in the third story, over a hundred patients; but between him and C. it must be done. Just as the lights were in full blaze, one poor fellow went to heaven; he looked up so scared and then lay back dead. Another one died before morning.

After the lights were out, the doctor, with the crowd generally who had collected around the hospital, composed of artisans, navy officers, niggers who were impressed with a guard to be made to sing, and all nicely drunk, started on a lark. They went all over town, screaming and shouting, came back to the hospital about twelve, woke up all the patients, then went to Mrs. Palmer's, who was alone with K., and scared her out of her life, came back at one again, and had another row. Finally, the officer of the day came and told them he knew his duty and would perform it. They were for fighting him; but someone was wise enough to advise them to go home; so at last we had peace.

I don't know how late it was when he arose. I did not see him till morning, when he borrowed my key to the store-room. I sent it by the boy; and when I went for it, he had given it to C. with orders not to let me have it again. My own key! I went right to C. and took it from him. I told him not to dare to refuse it. Of course, he gave it up, for he knew what Dr. Palmer would say; but he wanted so much to keep it. I should like to see anyone get it again but Dr. Palmer.

Now comes the news, through him, that Doctor is not coming back and that we are to have a new surgeon-in-charge. I am in despair. The impression is that Dr. Palmer is to have a hospital at Wilmington, where he is now. If he is not to return, you will have the pleasure of soon seeing me at home, for my experience with Dr. M. has quite sickened me of hospitals. I have had such good surgeons since the first, and have been always so respected that it is hard now to get a bad one.

Now you know I am an old grumbler and are disgusted with me; but I have not told you nearly all; enough, however, to let you see how hateful this week has been.

Did I tell you about General Meigs coming here to see me, and how polite he was? Well, he did. Miss Dix, his partner and friend, had recommended me so highly, and he saw our need of a bathroom and of various other things. After he had written the order for these, he turned to me and said:

"Madam, they have to thank you for anything that is done for this hospital. Miss Dix's high recommendation of you alone brought me here; tell me if there is anything else I can do for you."

Think of a live general, with stars and all, saying that to me! I bet I felt proud!

Beaufort, April 21, Sunday ("I guess").
I would rather be in bed tonight than writing letters, for I am cold as ice and so tired; it has been a miserable kind of day; it took so long to get through my wards, and then I have so many little things to see to. My old habit of playing off Sunday won't do now; I never get any time, and after all is done so many want letters written that I never have a moment in my room. All my leisure today has been spent in packing, for I don't know what moment Doctor may send for me. Dr. Palmer, I mean; and I want to be ready when his summons comes. I am so impatient to be off.

He wants all the old hands he can get; he has a thousand patients by this, and only green hands, besides C., and W., the chief clerk. I think Dr. Salter was real good to give them up, but he is such a true friend to the doctor. God knows what would have become of us during the M. reign if he had not come to help us out. I shall sometime tell you all about that terrible time. I feel too indignant now to talk about it, but I'm more down on whiskey than ever.

This has been a long week, though I have had so much to do. They have at last fitted up my linen room, and we had a large requisition of clothes come, and I have just made order there.

It is a job to lift and pack this heavy linen, but it pays; for on inspection they all admire the order there. We got a splendid woman in charge of the low diet, a Mrs. Bickerdyke. (See Mary A. Livermore's *My Story of the War.*) She began with the war, knows all about cooking, and can cook forty things at once. I never saw such a worker; she stirs round the cook-house with a big meat fork or ladle upraised, and looks as if she would annihilate them all; but there is no more pilfering; the sick men get all their dues while she is around.

Yesterday one of the cooks stole a custard pudding, and, though she had a dozen others, she missed it at once, and stormed around till she found it. Then she turned on him; when he said he laid it aside for a sick officer, he "got it,"—first for the lie and then for the steal. She knows all the celebrities, had charge of the Western and Southern departments, knows Sherman well and Grant too; has many notes from both. She is the most independent woman I ever knew; altogether she is a character. Miss Dix likes her very much and urged her coming here at once. She goes to Smithville as soon as she gets this shebang running right.

It is so lonely here I could not stand it long, especially with the terrible calamity that has be fallen us (Lincoln's assassination); I can think of nothing else. Today is the first paper I have seen with any account of it, one of the 17th. The only comfort I have, when any calamity comes, is in remembering Gustav's words: "Now be sure, my Molly, Heaven helps;" and out of this may come some great good. The sacrifice of such a true, good man may be necessary to show the world how bad the South is; and, then, he was perhaps too much a Christian gentleman to deal justly with such men. Oh, dear, when will the end come and what will it be? I begin so to long for peace and to be at home.

Beaufort, April 30 (1865).

This has been such a long, anxious week, waiting for a summons from Dr. Palmer, and every moment expecting to leave. You see, in anticipation of my leaving soon, they sent all my wounded men North on Tuesday, and I had not even the comfort of taking care of them. Lord knows, though, I have had work enough to do. I have just had shelves put in the linen room and had order to make there, besides crowding two weeks washing into one, which has been hard work, for I have not half help enough. With all the niggers here, I can't get enough to do the washing. I must be there nearly all my time to keep what I have at the tubs. For all this I thought the week would never end. I packed almost everything the first of the week, and every day want something which, of course, lies at the very bottom of the trunk.

The guns from the fort in memory of Lincoln were sad enough; every half hour their solemn booming came to us, and everyone seemed so impressed by them. There has been some demonstration in this miserable, dirty little town, a black rag now and then; but the show is very scarce.

The town is cram-jam full of returned Secesh, all swelling about in their uniforms, swaggering as usual, saying the South is not beaten yet, it is just unlooked-for circumstances that have brought her where she is. Wouldn't you think they had had enough by this time? There are rows every day among the returned and our soldiers. I hate the very sight of them.

I had a time this morning with one of the women. Once a month she has had a series of hysteric fits, and the last time they lasted a fortnight, with constant doctoring and some other of the women always to watch her. I did not know the trick, and when they came on yesterday, I began again, till Doctor told me she was really as well as I; if she had been whipped out of the first one, she would never have had a second.

So, when they came this morning saying that Dorcas was dying, could not speak, etc., I rushed up and, first thing, gave her ears a rousing slap; then a real good shaking was administered, accompanied by a right smart scolding. She soon winked her eyes (it's wonderful how long she could hold them open), and then she began to cry like any other nigger; so, I administered another dose of each, topped off with a dose (full strength) of *asafoetida*, turpentine *ile*, and some other nauseous *pizen* mixtures.

The girls all stood around crying, thinking it was too bad. I asked them what for; they said they could not help taking on so. If I'd been big enough and strong enough, I would have slapped them all; as it was, I shut them all out of the room and left Miss Dorcas alone, with orders for no one to approach her under pain of immediate dismissal from the hospital. When I went there at noon, my lady was up, in full feather, eating a hearty dinner of beans and pork; so now I understand treating hysteria as well as wounds.

I have such a funny little man for a page. He is a Second Massachusetts man, and was in Chattanooga, Atlanta, and Nashville, being one of the July recruits. He is a Russian, and had been only three days in the country when he enlisted. He says "he fight for freedom," was probably a serf (though he says not), and is certainly a Jew. He is the only second man we have ever had here, so I claimed him right off; as he is a tailor, I had need of him in the linen room. Last week he got tired of mending, and said: "Lookee here, I can find work to do, silk dresses make, all lady's work do; I am woman tailor in mine country. Can I not make you dress?" I remembered my long-talked-of double silk-muslin dress; so, gave him the materials, and my black calico for a pattern, locked him in my room, and left him to his fate.

Before the next evening he had everything completed, and much better than I could have done,—even trimmed with black silk. I was in ecstasies, and sent Uncle Massachusetts (my other old man) up to town to buy me a calico. He brought me back a flaming pink one, saying he knew I liked pink, for I always had pink roses in my waist. That was made in a jiffy. Then I gave him my old purple calico to cut over, and so on, until he has repaired and made over every dress I had. Everything is in complete order for summer; he can wash and iron those that needed it; I never saw such a useful man.

When I am in the room, he amuses me so with his talk, half German and half broken English, with now and then a Russian word that makes me expect to see his head come off, it sounds so hard. Sometimes he says, "Shall I tell you a story die Bublee (Bible)?" So, he begins to chatter about Pharaoh and Moses, particularly Joseph and the other old fellow and that naughty wife of his. He is so quaint and in earnest that you can't but be interested; anyway, in one week he has done more than I should in a year.

He lives in Boston, and we will all have him sew for us when we get home. He says he has a "gal," but she is too cross and too old for him, only she has his four hundred and fifty dollars bounty money and he must marry her to get it. "Then I guess I run away." He doesn't know anybody in the regiment, only his captain, *Fellen*, he calls him; I don't know who he is. He was sent back to the hospital from Alexandria, and his legs are so short he could only march as far as Goldsboro' and was again sent back; he is invaluable to me. I am to take him to Smithville when I go, if I ever do.

We were mustered today, probably for the last time for most of us. I shall stay until the last gun fires if there is anything for me to do. Did I tell you about Mrs. Bickerdyke, who has come down here from the Western army and is cooking for this hospital? She is perfectly splendid. To be sure, she snubs me and everybody else; but, Lord, how she works, and what good things she makes; our men are better fed now than they would be at home, even the best of them.

She has many stores of her own, fruits, etc., but those are nothing to her cooking of the common food; she talks bad grammar and jaws us all, but I don't care; her heart is the best, and she will make most every soldier live, and how she hates a Reb! She is never afraid of anyone. Once old Dr. S., of Alexandria, was around inspecting her kitchen, drunk. He found fault with everything; she took him by the nape of the neck, led him out, called a guard, and told them to take this drunken man to headquarters and she would have him court-martialled. He was afterwards glad enough to apologise and to get out of that place, or she would have done it, sure.

Tonight the rumour has come that Booth is killed and taken to Washington; somebody saw somebody who said he saw a paper,—that is the way we get all the news; if it is true, it is too good a death. I would have liked to boil him in my boilers over a slow fire, or to have my girls chop him up in the chopping-tray.

Beaufort, Wednesday.

I was so unexpectedly pleased last night at C.'s appearance; he came down to take me to Smithville; we leave here today at noon by cars to Goldsboro , etc. They have about seven hundred patients at Smithville. C. says it's a pleasant, clean town. The worst is there are three other nurses there! It will be rather funny moving four boxes, two trunks, two chairs, and a table, two dorgs (mine and Doctor's), looking-glass, and Jack (the Russian) with his knapsack; he is the guardian angel over all. I asked him to do something for me last night; he said, "I do anything for you; when you tell me, I fall down dead in the water," meaning, throw himself overboard.

Smithville, May 14 (1865).

At last I am here where I have so longed to be. We left Beaufort Wednesday afternoon, at five, in the cars. I was at last really on the way, seated in a box-car with all my boxes about me. They told us we should have a hard journey, so I was prepared for anything we might encounter. There was no passenger car on the route, and this had been especially used for transporting sick and wounded from the front; so, the lice and fleas! to say nothing of the dirty straw with which it was filled. We rode all night. There were five in our party, and a number of drunken officers, some of whom were Rebels, so the ride was not the most agreeable in the world. Everybody was lying round on the straw; there was not a seat excepting the trunks and boxes. The first misfortune was that C. let my mocking bird loose; I could have cried, only that he was so sorry.

About seven in the morning we arrived at Goldsboro'; it is a pretty town and very little affected by the war; everything seemed intact but the fences; those are mostly gone. We had no time to go to the hotel for breakfast, as the quartermaster said the train would leave immediately; so I ran into the first house and asked the woman, whose breakfast was on the table, for a cup of coffee. She gave it willingly, but she was rabid Secesh and kept talking about the troubles she had seen.

After all our hurry, we did not leave here till ten. We sat there on a platform car in the hot sun till I thought I should bake. I was so glad to get started again. The cars were crowded with returning Rebels, full of discontent with "Yanks," but glad the war was over and to get home. Some of them talked real saucy; but I quickly shut them up. It was five o'clock when we got to Wilmington. The country is lovely in some parts,—perhaps not really so, but it is so long since I have seen green fields and woods. You would hardly have known us for smut and dust when we arrived.

I had hardly got bathed and brushed when in came Dr. Barnes. He had a message in his pocket, just received from Dr. Palmer. He (Dr. Barnes) had telegraphed to Dr. Palmer:

"Is Mary von Olnhausen with you? If so, can you spare her to go to Raleigh?"

Dr. Palmer's answer was:

"Not here, but expected every moment; can't spare her."

He was for taking me off without more words, as he has eight hundred sick and wounded there, and no nurse. If I had been going to anyone else but Dr. Palmer, I would not have hesitated; but I knew it would disappoint him so much.

Dr. Barnes went from me to General Abbott. In talking of the war, Mrs. Abbott said, "Doctor, have you ever met Mrs. von Olnhausen?"

"I have just left her," said the doctor; so in ten minutes he was back with the general, who would not hear an excuse, but took me off to his quarters. They are quite splendid, and I had such a warm welcome from his wife (I told you I knew them in Manchester), and such a pleasant visit with them. Next morning the captain sent for me as the boat was starting. General Abbott sent word that the lady had not breakfasted, and that the boat must be delayed till she came on board,—so much for being a general's guest.

The sail down is very nice and of much interest; the river is full of obstructions, with many sunken boats; they think the torpedoes are about all out of it. The forts, all except Fisher and Caswell, are already dismantled and their banks are crumbling. Indeed, I was surprised, all the way through, to see so few traces of such recent fighting.

My ward is a large one,—over sixty beds, all with wounded; it's not quite completed. Yesterday and today I have been helping generally, and need enough there is of help. One thing I did which I suppose you will all be shocked at, though the patients have been too glad. I shot three big pigs from the cook-house door,—one at the first shot and two at the last. We could not lay a thing down that they did not devour. They would come right up to the tents or cook-house; nobody would take them, and it required all of us to keep them away.

I said I'd shoot them and take the consequences if they would bring me a gun; so, when the gun was brought, I was bound to do it. The most I have to boast is that I shot them all through the heart. Doctor has appointed me chief huntsman, and the patients had a bully dinner, and, more than all, I think the Rebels will have a wholesome fear of me when I meet them with a weapon in my hands.

I long to be settled down to work and to have the thing fairly running; but it takes so long to start a new hospital. Moreover, every one now seems indifferent; you can't make him work. All they think of is getting home. For myself, I wait patiently till it is all over; this hospital undoubtedly will be the last to be broken up, and I shall stay, at least, till Dr. Palmer goes. This is a most dilapidated town, right opposite Fort Caswell, and with a fort in its very centre. Doctor's house is close by it and a quarter of a mile from the camp, so it is quite a walk through the sand. I hope soon to be nearer. Last night I took a horseback ride of about three miles; we passed many redoubts and rifle-pits, but all in disuse now. It is such a sandy, uninteresting country all around here; but any country is better than none, so I enjoyed the ride.

Smithville, May 21 (1865).

What do you say that I did not write my usual Sunday letter; were you mad as a pig? Well, you would have been if you had had as bad a stomach-ache as I did all day. I never did have a worse one. If I'd had courage to write the letter, it would have been a succession of faces such as only I can make, varied with interjections that you don't like to hear. As to writing Monday and Tuesday, or any other day this week, it has simply been impossible. I have had all I could do early and late to get clothes enough washed to have the men clean by Saturday night. The clothing has been neglected, was scattered everywhere, and was so abused.

My house is all done, so now I can tell you about it. Perhaps if I had written a true account last Sunday you would have felt that it was about time to leave the army and retire to private life. I certainly felt so nearly all that week; it seemed impossible that order ever could come. I thought by being at the camp I could expedite matters, as I saw no prospect of a laundry or ward while I was a quarter of a mile off and the sand so deep it was killing us to walk it so many times a day. So, the doctor had a bed temporarily put up in the light-diet cook's pas—age-way (the only spare place he could find), while he hunted up quarters. Now there was an agreeable situation, from five in the morning a constant stream of darkies and cooks passing through, for it was the only store-room. I could not rise, of course, till one of the women gave me a chance to dress in her room.

Doctor finally found a house that would do for linen room and my quarters, using a big tent for laundry. It was the very best he could do, unless he went far from camp; but such a forlorn, dirty, tumble-down old hole you never saw in the North. Anything to get a house; so, by Wednesday I had my room ready and fell asleep in it. Luckily the lamp was burning, for I felt afraid to sleep there in the dark alone. Something wakened me after an hour or so; and on opening my eyes I saw the biggest kind of a rat gnawing a piece of candle on a stand at my side, and another in the corner of the window apparently ready to charge on me if I made a move.

I felt perfectly faint with terror; there are no windows in the house, only wooden shutters. I screamed to Jack as loud as I could, as if the poor soul could hear me; he sleeps in the work room, which, as usual, is some way from the house. No Jack came; but the noise I made scared the rats and they walked leisurely away, taking the candle with them (the piece, I mean). I sat up in bed and, happening to look at the wall, how can I describe the bedbugs! They were swarming from every crack and hole; they were countless. How the rest of that night was passed you may guess.

The next day I was back in the diet-cook's passage again. I liked the men best of the three. Then I began charging on the beasts with hot water by gallons, with mercurial ointment, and after that with two coats of whitewash, and with carpenters and chloride of lime for the rats. I got back again Wednesday and can for a while sleep comfortably. The house is cleaned and whitened and made close from top to bottom, and it really looks quite jolly. I have all my traps about my little room, and the doctor confiscated a bureau and a settee for me; so I am proud.

Jack has taken a little room nearer to me, one that I used for a soiled-clothes room. What could I do without the dear soul? He is just as devoted as one can be. He heard the orders read for all Sherman's men to go to Washington to be mustered out; for a little while he was delighted, got his knapsack ready, and danced round. I did not say a word against it, (how could I?) but I felt real bad. In about an hour I missed him; he came back directly clapping his hands and saying, "I no go, I no leave you; I tell Dr. Palmer and he say I stay."

Dr. Palmer reports that Jack came with eyes full of tears and said: "Doctor, I can no leave Mrs. O. I fall down dead before I leave her. I love her like my mother." Doctor was much amused with his devotion, and told him he could stay as long as he would. He is always doing something for my comfort, in such a funny way too. My bird and dog are his especial delight. He makes no friends excepting them. Altogether he is a character of my army experience.

This is certainly the strangest part, if not the hardest; and yet I really have enjoyed being here ten times as much as in Beaufort. I would not change for anything. I have the care of twenty washerwomen; a great care it is, too, and with such an amount of back washing to make up. My ward is ready for me now. I have about thirty wounded, but I can tell you more about them in my next, as I've seen them only now and then.

We have about four hundred patients here, mostly recruits and bummers. I never saw such an uninteresting set of men, all homesick and good for nothing, wanting simply to get home. It seems only a certain portion after all are to be mustered out. I don't know what these fellows who must stay will do. I thought, of course, all Sherman's army were going home.

My letter is more than usually stupid, but I am undergoing such a biting from the fleas I can hardly write. The other day I could not stand it a moment longer, rushed into my room and went hunting; the result was thirty fleas, the biggest louse you ever saw, and in the covering of my hoop-skirt an enormous bed-bug had built her nest and laid her eggs,—fairly domesticated herself and seemed settled for the summer. What do you think of that? North Carolina forever!

Smithville, Sunday, June 4, 1865.

I have my little shebang and laundry in perfect order. The tent for washing is the best in the land, and my hut, white inside and out, is too lovely for anything; and I can have a clean spread on the floor every day, since I control the wash. The whole arrangement is much better here than elsewhere. None of the women live on the land; they draw their rations every Saturday for the week. I give them Saturday afternoons and pay them all off before they leave. They have a dollar and fifty cents a week. I have four white women and fourteen *nigs*; if they stay away for half a day, I cut them down, so I have to call the roll twice a day. It makes me a heap of trouble; but I am sure of the work, and as there are no sevens or nines in the figures I get on amazingly well.

Two of my men are Rebels, mortally wounded, one through the lungs. The other has had a resection of the upper third of the left arm done by a Rebel surgeon, and done accordingly; he forgot to look and see that the elbow joint was shattered. I have so little patience with these surgeons. One of my boys was a prisoner in Andersonville several months; his limbs are full of scurvy scars. He is now wounded in the foot; he says he has never had enough to eat, and has that gnawing at his stomach all the time, no matter how many rations he gets. It is a real disease with so many of them. Another poor fellow was eleven months a prisoner for refusing to work in the fortifications about Richmond; they knocked him down, stamped on him, broke four of his ribs, and kicked his front teeth out.

He said to them, "Do all you can, but I'll never work on a breastwork or fortification for you to kill one of my own men from." They tried starving, and finally brought him to that horrid Salisbury, wounded and worn, and left him without shelter till both of his feet were frozen to the knees. Luckily some comrade got ice water and bathed them till the frost was out or he would have lost them both, as so many did. He is to me such a hero, but after all he suffered he says nothing was as bad as the hunger. He says about a thousand consented to work; those were better fed just to tantalize those who would not. He is a handsome little fellow as well as brave.

The medical director says this hospital will remain here all summer at any rate, so I suppose there is no chance of coming home at present, and it seems not well to go for a furlough when probably the fall will see us all at home.

I hear all the pickets are to be drawn in tomorrow. I am so glad; it will be nice to be able to walk out in the country again without being obliged to run for a pass. It is a long time since I have had that privilege. You can't make eyes at pickets; they just won't let one go past. Only the Massachusetts Second H. A. would, about Morehead. They knew me, and used to say, "When I go back on my beat, you just slip by."

Smithville, Sunday night, 12 o'clock.
This last week has been hateful. I wrote you that a brigade of soldiers were coming; well, sure enough, they came, and a greater set of scalawags never lived. I never heard of such men; they broke into houses, smashed ever so many heads, insulted women, stole horses and everything else they could steal, even went into Dr. Palmer's stable and carried off one of his horses. They were drunk and rowing all the time, and everyone had to go armed. I had Doctor's double-barrelled gun by my bed, and

only that I was smart enough to have shot those pigs I think I had been attacked, sure; for a lot of them came into the yard one night. Then one of them said, "You better let her be, she'll shoot you, and she can shoot, too, for I see her shoot three times and kill every pop." He did not say it was pigs I popped, so I guess they thought it was men. They went off growling and vowing they would kill my dog, who was barking furiously. What a dog that is! His horror is a *nig* or a Reb; one cannot come into the yard when he is unchained.

Smithville, June, Sunday.
Thursday, I went to Fort Fisher with Doctor and his family and some others; and that was truly a most delightful day, though the thermometer was nearly out of sight and the sand ankle deep; but the cool sea breezes were delightful, and, then, it is probably the greatest battlefield in America, and the first I have ever been on except New Berne, and there every trace had disappeared. But here all was so fresh and so wonderful to see. I wish I could describe the fort or even give you a faint idea of the work our men had before them.

The long unsheltered road they came down in the face of such a terrific fire seems too much for any stout hearts (they landed up the beach two miles); and the rushing forward of the hundred and fifty forlorn hope, all volunteers and armed with only axes to cut away the stockade to make an entrance for the troops (which the fire from the gunboats had failed to do) was perfectly heroic. Besides the sharpshooters at the stockade, stationed so closely with loop-holes to fire from, there were rows of rifle-pits to receive them if they succeeded, and the constant shower of shot and shell of all kinds. It's wonderful how one lived to strike a blow, and yet it was done, though almost all fell.

Friday.
There is the greatest excitement here over a tent fly that was missing. Some circumstances led Doctor to believe that one of the "first nine" in town (a pilot who has made "whips" of money during the war in the blockade runners) had it, as he was seen often talking with a hospital scalawag. So, Wednesday night, the doctor called and told him he was informed he had a fly belonging to the government. He swore as a gentleman and also by a solemn oath "on the square" as a man, that he hadn't

it or any hospital property.

Doctor told him he was sorry to proceed farther, but he must, circumstances pointed him out so plainly, and gave him his choice,—to permit him and his stewards quietly to search or to have the provost guard. T. tried all arguments and, finding the doctor determined, said he thought he could tell him where some of them were. So, he told of a man in the country who had two. He thought surely then the doctor would go off. Not so.

Doctor said, "Come, take your choice."

"Well, Doctor, if you won't betray me, perhaps I can find two of them;" so he went upstairs and brought them down. Doctor had missed only one. Then T. said he bought them of that bad man for five dollars each,—such a lie! The first cost of one is about seventy dollars, and these are of the very best duck. Doctor went right off, got a guard, and searched the house; it was eleven at night, and the man's wife, Mary, was in bed. When they went into her room, he said, "Don't be alarmed, Mary, cover up your head, these rude men shan't hurt you." Such a homely, snuff-chewing thing you never saw; if he had anything else, it was under Mary, and Doctor was too foolishly polite to search her bed.

Well, all this developed other things; so, they commenced yesterday morning and searched every house in town, and it was truly wonderful what they found. Not a single house where there was not something,—quantities of bed linen, guns, three new flags, crockery, buckets, tinware, even hospital slippers. The boys had lots of fun out of it. Nobody knew how anything came in the house; "Why, it had been there years before the Yanks came." The fools could not read, and there was the hospital mark on everything!

Anyway, this is the worst set of soldiers ever did live, all recruits and bounty jumpers who steal everything and sell it again for a trifle. The richest man in town, whose wife is just going North for a summer tour, after her four years' imprisonment, had a quantity of linen spreads that they were using for table-cloths. She "had not the least idea how they came in the house." A guard has gone into the country today expecting to make a great haul, having heard of a lot of things that were seen out there.

Doctor is almost discouraged; everything seems to happen down here in Smithville; of all the places, I've been in yet it is the meanest. It might be so pretty, too, and is, indeed, now. The crepe-myrtle grows here like the lilacs at home, only much larger; but every house has many trees of it, and the beautiful china pink of the blossom against the rich live-oak foliage is perfectly lovely. One peculiarity of the town is its thousand swings, sometimes as many as three or four in a yard. Everybody swings, *nigs* and whites; these moonlight nights everyone is flying through the air. Dr. Curtis says it is only since the war that it has become a feature of the place. I guess the ropes have washed in from the wrecks of the blockade runners.

The town is full of returned Rebels who are insolent as they dare to be,—excepting those who have been prisoners; those all say they have been treated as well as if they had been one of us and are, consequently, a shade more polite; but the spirit of secession is not laid yet. Can you believe that many of them still think slavery will be re-established? Can one have a stronger proof of their ignorance? Imagine these millions of men who have been fighting for their freedom brought back to chains again!

Five hundred sick and wounded coloured soldiers have been admitted since I wrote, all waiting to be discharged. They are many of them of the Second Maryland, the first regiment of blacks that I ever saw, on their march through Alexandria. They are a splendid set of men, have always been at the front, and are so much better disciplined than the white soldiers who are here. One who stands guard at my house has had five bullets through him, and yet has lost only three months and never had a furlough; he is such a manly fellow, says his old father in Baltimore told him and his two brothers never to come back to him unless they had proved themselves true soldiers and good men.

Smithville, August 28 (1865).

My two little pet birds are devoured by wretches of cats, and this morning my only other mocking bird was dead in his cage. I am so mad, as now I have only the two cats and the redbird; I hope these will live until I get home. I feel impatient to be off, have commenced packing, and am having everything washed, wearing all my cast-offs so as to be ready at a moment's notice.

I don't expect to get off this week, but will the first of next.
We are sending the patients away as fast as we can, and they are already reduced to fifty, so my cares are very light. As I have only a few women to look after, I have time to repair breaks, etc. How I'm longing to see you and hoping to have a letter; that is my best comfort. Soon you won't have my scribble to decipher, but will have me chattering. I shall be a change, at least.

This was the last letter from the Civil War. How highly valued were the services that she had given to the soldiers during these three years and more is made plain by the following letter from the last surgeon under whom she served, Dr. Palmer, a letter heartily endorsed by Medical Director Hand and Major-General Palmer. It is addressed to her brother-in-law.

U. S. A. Gen'l Hospital,
Smithville, N. C., July 4, 1865.

Sir,—I have recently received from the office of the Surgeon General, U. S. A., a Circular Order, directing me to forward to him "the names of those ladies who have rendered valuable services, gratuitously, for more than three years past, in attendance upon sick and wounded soldiers in hospitals."
This order was designed, I suppose, to secure some public and striking recognition of the services alluded to. I think this is right.
But there is a class of ladies who have rendered extremely valuable services to the sick and wounded Union soldiers in hospitals, but who do not come within the terms of the order above mentioned. The Volunteer Nurses, who worked under the supervision of Miss Dix, received, from the Government, twelve dollars per month. Many of these women were so self-sacrificing and faithful and efficient, that we who live to enjoy Freedom a second time won, and, I hope *forever* won, can scarcely manifest, adequately, our gratitude to these women.
And among all the female nurses whom I have known or heard of, not one is better entitled to eminent and substantial notice than is Mrs. Mary Von Olnhausen of Lexington, Mass.
From my own observation, and from the statements of our lamented friend, Surg. J. B. Bellangee, I conclude that the services rendered by this lady to the sick and wounded soldiers, and thus

to the Government, and to us all, have been quite equal in value to those afforded by any other person in her sphere of labour.

Her whole soul has been in the work. She very early acquired a marvellous dexterity in the management of the wounded. Thus, with her wonderful physical endurance, she was able to do more good than any nurse I ever knew. She was literally untiring in her labours. By her zeal and usefulness and general deportment, she entitled herself to the respect of us all.

Soldiers who owe their lives to her care and skilful attention are scattered, now, over nearly all the Northern States. They will remember her with gratitude. I presume that is all she will wish for. I suspect that Mrs. Von Olnhausen is not ambitious for notoriety or fame. But I take the liberty to suggest that the citizens of Massachusetts may with propriety, and honour to themselves, offer to Mrs. V. O. some substantial testimonial, which shall manifest their appreciation of her services and at the same time do her good. She is in every way entitled to all she will receive, and ought to feel no delicacy in accepting it.

This statement of mine is prompted in part, by hearing that the friends of Mrs. George, a female nurse, who "died at her post" in Wilmington a short time since, had purchased, for presentation to her, a home in the State in which she had been a resident. To me this was suggestive. A fee simple, in a piece of land, is worth a thousand golden trinkets.

I suppose you know Mrs. V. O. and are her friend. So, without apology for writing to a stranger, I simply hope that you and her other friends may sometime act upon the suggestion given. I know many whom you will never see who will gladly take part with you. Yours respectfully,

J. M. Palmer,
Surg. 3rd N.Y.V. in Charge Hosp.

Endorsed:

Med. Dir.'s Office,
Newburn, N. C., July 17, 1865.

Mrs. M. Von Olnhausen has served in hospitals under my direction for nearly two years past, and I take pleasure in endorsing all the statements of Surg. Palmer. This lady has won the respect and confidence of all brought in contact with her; and by her devotion to the sick and wounded soldiers has deserved all a grateful country can do for her.

D. W. Hand,
Colonel and Med. Dir, Dept. N. C.

August 2, 1865.

I most cheerfully endorse all that has been said herein of Mrs.
Von Olnhausen. I believe that this lady has done more good
in the hospitals than any other female nurse I ever saw or of
whom I have ever heard.

I. N. Palmer,
Bt. Maj. Genl. U. S. A. (late Comdg. Dept. of N. C.).

A more formal and more general testimonial of the value of her
services follows. Signed, as it is, by Governor Andrew and other State
officials, it is in a measure a definite recognition by Massachusetts of
the good she had done in the cause of that State and of the Union.
This testimonial would have proved of the highest value to her five
years later had it not been for a misfortune involving it, which will
later appear.

Admitting as we do, that the noble and patriotic devotion of
the Soldier has not been fully appreciated, we feel that the devoted service of the truly *patriotic women*, who have served so
faithfully at the bedside of the sick and wounded in camp and
hospital, demand of us our most profound gratitude.

That although we have no fear that History will fail to do full
justice to this noble band of *patriots*, yet in many cases those
who have received kind attention, and the friends of such, cannot be satisfied without some more substantial manifestation.

In no case can a proper manifestation be more deserving than
to Mrs. Von Olnhausen, than whom no one has been more
self-sacrificing, no one has laboured with more success or with
a more honest purpose.

We are therefore most happy to have this opportunity to make
manifest in some slight manner our feeling and regard for the
truly noble and *patriotic character* of her we are truly proud to
call our Friend.

(Signed)   J. M. Palmer,
Surg. 3rd N. Y. Vols. formerly in charge of U. S. A. Gen. Hospitals
"Mansfield" and "Smithville," N. C.

John A. Andrew,
Governor of Massachusetts.

WM. Schouler,
>Adj. General of Mass.

WM. I. Dale,
>Surgeon–General of Massachusetts.

Nehemiah Brown,
>A. A. G. of Mass.

John Cummings, Jr.

I. H. Spring.

H. L. Simonds.

Chas. Choate.

Frank Wrisley.

Anson P. Hooker,
>Asst. Surg. Genl. Mass.

WM. C. Capelle,
>Capt. Mil. Asst. to Surg. Genl. Mass.

Josiah Bartlett, M. D.

Henry I. Bowditch, M. D.

W. T. Mcalpine,
>1st Lieut. 2nd Mass. Infty.

James Vila.

Edward Whitney.

Chapter 8

Scarcely had Mrs. von Olnhausen recovered from the fatigues of her Civil War campaign than she determined again to take up the more difficult, because more monotonous, duties of life on the Illinois prairie. During her three years absence, her brother's wife had died, leaving, besides the four other children, an infant boy.

This second experience of the Western prairies was far harder than the first, and was probably the most "strenuous" period of this active and unusual life. To bring up a baby, to control four other children, to cook, sew, wash, and mend for a large family, is far from easy under the best of conditions; to do all this under the hard circumstances of frontier life is appalling. But Mary von Olnhausen could extract sunshine out of the sourest cucumbers, and the very hardships of her life were made sources of simple pleasures for herself and the children of whom she took such admirable care.

The long journey to the "timber" to get the winter's wood became, under her management, a pleasure excursion; the planting and the harvesting, when neighbour A must borrow all neighbour B's family and men, and must, in turn, send all his family and men to B's, became a bustling picnic-time, the sixteen hungry extra men to be fed making her already busy hands but fly the faster. The good years, when there was an abundant crop but no market, and the bad years, when there was a good market but no crops, would seem to have been equally disheartening; but they never discouraged her.

Always she was seeking, and her optimistic, childlike nature was ever finding the beautiful, where others would have seen only the dreary and the squalid in the nature and the human nature of that monotonous, semi-civilized prairie-land. Possessed of a keen sense of humour, she extracted the last possible drop of enjoyment from the eccentricities and idiosyncrasies of that extraordinary folk which, dazzled by the richness of the new soil and the glamour of frontier life, had drifted into her neighbourhood from every corner of the United States.

With what unction she used to tell of the woman who, in the neighbourhood prayer-meeting, thanked God that she had had a change of heart on "Tuesday, at three, by Mr. Phinney's clock;" of the relatives from far and wide who came to the funeral of one of her brother's hired men and camped in his house, as was the prairie custom, for three weeks; of the extraordinary sayings and doings of a neighbouring family of poor whites who exhibited amazingly the primitive instincts of the untutored and unmoral mind. In her failure to record these experiences we have lost what would have been a distinct contribution to the social history of the middle West.

In the summer of 1870 came news of the Franco-Prussian War. Mrs. von Olnhausen was immediately fired with a wish to go, being inspired both with professional zeal and with ambition to be of service to her husband's countrymen. She had never been abroad; with a good knowledge of French, she had almost none of German; she was aware that every difficulty would be put in the way of foreign nurses; she had no money, and none of that held by the German organisations of America was available for such a use as this. But she begged sufficient funds from her friends; secured, as was easy, letters from those who were competent to speak of her services in the Civil War, (see note below); began vigorously to study German; and in October of 1870 set sail for Liverpool.

★★★★★★

Commonwealth of Massachusetts.
Office of Surgeon General.
Boston, October 17, 1870.

It gives me pleasure to state, that the bearer, Mrs. Mary Von Olnhausen of Massachusetts, United States of America, recently of the State of Illinois, distinguished herself during the late war by her devotion to our sick and wounded soldiers.

So continuous and disinterested was her humane service, that by direction of the late Governor Andrew of Massachusetts, a letter of thanks was addressed her by this Department, and she is cordially recommended to the consideration and courtesy of all engaged in ameliorating the hardships of war, now present abroad.

WM. I. Dale,

Surgeon-General of Massachusetts.
American Association for Relief of Misery of
Battlefields, New York.

New York, Bible House,
October 21, 1870.

I desire heartily to commend Mrs. Olnhausen, the bearer of this letter, to all the officers and friends of the International Association for the Relief of Sick and Wounded Soldiers, in Europe, as a woman of great worth, devotion, and experience, meriting the full confidence and respect of all who value self-sacrifice, patient and persistent labour in the humblest details of service to suffering humanity. She goes to offer her services to the sick and wounded, and any who can aid her in getting to work in this blessed business, will merit the blessing of God and the friends of humanity.

Henry W. Bellows,
President of the American Branch of
the International Asso. for Relief, etc.

★★★★★★

Thence she made her way without difficulty to Berlin, and, after the red tape inseparable from war-time, secured permission to go to the front, which, then, was not far from Paris. But, on her way from Berlin to the seat of war, a misfortune of the worst sort befell her in the loss of her only trunk, containing all her letters and credentials, and all her clothing excepting what she wore. Her supply of money failing to cover any such contingency as this, she really suffered throughout the campaign for lack of warm clothes; and the loss of her credentials, of course, gave her endless trouble.

She wrote not a word of this, however, to her friends in America; and they knew nothing of her loss and her discomforts from this source until the following March. Then came letters from the Consul at Nancy announcing that an unclaimed trunk containing letters and luggage, which he described, had lain there for many months. This misadventure accounts for many of the difficulties which Mrs. von Olnhausen was to experience, and explains the note of discouragement, so unusual with her, which runs through many of her foreign letters.

Leaving Berlin on the 10th of November, she stayed at Nancy five days, seeking the lost trunk. Thence she was forwarded, *via* Epernay, Reims, Thierry, and Meaux to Lagny (all this taking ten days), there to await orders from Versailles. But, though she waited more than three weeks and used every effort to be sent forward, she could secure neither the necessary permission nor the essential transportation. Finally, she determined to go back to Epernay to seek employment in the English ambulance there.

They, however, could give her no place, but sent her on to the ambulance at Metz, where she stayed only two days. Going thence to Orleans, armed with letters to American and English surgeons, she served for short periods in various ambulances, notably at Meung, until she found at last, in January, 1871, definite and established duties at Vendôme, upon the Loire, about midway between Orleans and Tours. Her letters and journal give, in far less detail than is to be wished, the chronicle of these difficult and discouraging wanderings.

> Victoria Hotel, Liverpool, Eng.,
> November 1, 1870.
>
> I'm here in the smokiest of towns, and so confused with the noise of landing that I hardly know myself. Mr. (Thomas) Hughes came to me this morning and asked to introduce himself. He said he had often wished to speak; but I seemed so absorbed in my German that he would not be intrusive. He spoke nicely of America, and gave me much pleasant information. We talked all the morning, and when we parted on the pier he gave me his card and made me promise, when I came through England, to send at once to him and he would show me everything in London worth seeing, and would even take me to Miss Nightingale, who, though a great invalid, will always see him; so, I felt quite proud. They all had supposed me some forlorn German *frau* who could speak no English, as they heard me speaking only to the German passengers. When they had known German themselves, they would soon have detected me. It's too funny how I dare blunder along as I do; but, after all, courage is the best, and it's not so hard as learning to wash. I start at one today with my Prussian officer, who speaks no English, and we shall have *drôle* times making mouths at each other. He has only three bird-cages and a parrot who talks continually, so imagine us *en route*.

> Berlin, November 4, 1870.
>
> At last I am in Berlin, where I have so long wished to be. This has been a day of pleasure. I am at a little hotel, second class.

Herr L., who wanted first to see his family and gladden his five children with his livestock, advised me to rest today; tomorrow he will come at eleven and take me to see Mr. Happ. So, after a bath and breakfast, I started out alone to see the town and air my German. It has been splendid. I hope I shall go again, but it's impossible to know till I see those I have to. I hope to be sent at once to the front.

Berlin, Thursday, November 10, 1870.
It seems a hundred days since I came here, I have seen and done so much. I am to go to Reims. I am sent to the Sanitary Association, who will put me at once where I wish to be. If I am not satisfied there, I am to be sent to any place I like.
It was a great favour, my going at all, as there are very strict orders for no one to be sent; but being an American and coming as I do with letters from Dr. Bellows and the others has helped. I must say I began to feel a little anxious, fearing I should never get off. In the meantime, I have spent most delightful days wandering about the city, which is truly beautiful. Wherever I saw people going in I went too; so, I have seen much.

Château Thierry, November 20, 1870.
After I had delivered my letters, one of which was to a Fraulein von somebody, I went to visit the two hospitals she has under her care, and no words can tell about them. In our most disorganised days in our worst field hospitals I saw nothing like it. The beds were abominable, the patients dirty and, it seemed to me, in every way uncomfortable. The rooms were not even ventilated, and I couldn't see that anybody was doing anything but eating and drinking; that seemed continuous. You would not believe me if I told you all she drank on one round right out of the bottle; I would have had to occupy one of the beds before the first half-hour. Her face was ruddy as the wine before we parted; every person we met she stopped to tell how much she had to do; and yet all that day she did nothing but talk, drink, and eat.
Twice we had coffee, and she always took out her little flask of brandy; "Sary Gamp" could not have liked it better. How "von" tells! Otherwise I think she would not stay long in the position. She went with me to the French woman's where I am billeted, and talked steadily in German, although neither understood

133

the other; it was very funny to hear them. The *Madame* fired the last shot by saying "Goodbye, lady of the Grand Nation. It is time you too were in Prussia with its three hundred and fifty thousand soldiers!"

There are no more letters extant covering the period of the next five weeks; but in place of letters we have the journal kept scrawlingly in a little black book. It begins with a pencilled itinerary, but is silent as to route and experiences from December 19, 1870, to March 30, 1871, that period being partly covered, however, by somewhat fragmentary letters. The dates in the diary are hopelessly confused, Mrs. von Olnhausen finding it difficult, throughout her life, to know which of her busy days was which.

Left New York 22nd. October, 1870.
Arrived 32nd October (? Nov. 1) , Liverpool.
Arrived 5th November, Berlin.
Left Berlin 10th November.
Arrived at Nancy 12th November.
Left Nancy 17th November.
Arrived at Épernay 17th November.
Left Épernay 18th November.
Arrived at Reims 18th November.
Left Reims 19th November.
Arrived at Château Thierry 19th November.

Château Thierry, November 20, 1870.
So dark and late and muddy when I got here that I was not prepared to see such a lovely town as it is. I had some difficulty in finding lodgement, but at last was housed. I wanted supper and wine. The people, at first, were cross and unwilling; but I took the high hand and let them know I *would* have it. After a while it went better, when they learned I was American; so, I had a good bed and the best of coffee; and, besides, they cleaned the mud from my clothes and shoes. One has to put on high airs with these people. When I got here, I found I must be delayed some days. The railroad is torn up to Meaux. This is so discouraging.

November 24, Meaux.
At last I am so far on my way. Dr. Schmidt gave me transportation with his colonel. I started in the *coupe* of a big wagon, in

charge of a friend of his. After a little the lieutenant of the command offered us his chaise. That was very nice; but my companion was very drunk from too much port wine, quarrelled with the officers, and drove over everything except the houses. So, at noon, when we halted, the lieutenant claimed his chaise and drove me the rest of the way to Meaux over the most beautiful road, smooth as a floor and lined with double rows of trees. Everywhere were lovely views and such picturesque villages. I was not at all tired, though we drove fifty miles.

I had a letter to Count Gleist, who, though it was so late, received me kindly, with promises to do all he could for me. He gave me such pleasant quarters with the nicest of French ladies. When she found I was American, she was so pleasant, gave me a nice dinner, and we sat till late talking,—really talking, though my French is very bad. She understood a little German, however. She has seen much suffering through all the wars, is a Bourbon, and does not believe it possible for France ever to become a Republic,—so also I. In the morning, I found such nice coffee and delicious bread and butter; and then went, by appointment, to Count Gleist. He promised to send me, during the day, to Lagny. Though it is winter, the flowers are blooming in the fields and gardens. The garden of old *Madame* is very fine, and her house is filled with flowers. She sits all day embroidering altarpieces. Her only son is a colonel at Paris.

November 25, Lagny.

It was quite dark when we left Meaux, but we were here by seven, and I was brought, by the count's direction, to the cloister. Just as I arrived came also some Protestant Sisters from Stuttgart, the freshest, nicest-looking girls, all eager to go to work. We had a very merry evening and slept in the large dormitory together. This was a boarding-school; but is now a hospital, as is every large house in the town. It is a very little place, with but few wounded in it. I did not expect to find them here; but this is another step. I have letters to Count P. with orders to send me farther. Always farther! When shall I come to the end? I have sent to him, and he will see me at one o'clock; so, I wait here in this dismal abode. It's raining hard and there is nothing to see; so, it's rather forlorn. An English doctor is here who offers to be my guide to the count.

Saturday (November 26).
I went with the English doctor to see Graf P., who promises to do all for me. I have such hateful quarters in a cloister. The Sisters are more than horrid to the "*Deutschers*," though they treat me a little better, being an American. I have no fire in my room except a foot-stove which carries me back to the days when I had such beautiful times in the old garret. I hate black bread; but they do make good coffee. This is the first day that I have lost courage; but it's impossible to feel jolly with stone walls all around and so cold. If I could have only one letter from home, I would feel quite happy; but so far, I have heard not one word since I left so long ago.

Sunday (November 27).
I went to church with the Mother, both forenoon and afternoon. It's such a ridiculous little church, rigged up with painted windows giving such an abominable light. After church, I took a long walk with the Mother through the town. This terrible war! The place is full of destruction: beautiful villas entirely destroyed; furniture, pictures, glass, all broken in pieces; trees and shrubs torn up; marble statues all in ruins. Every house not destroyed is occupied as a hospital or bureau. In one house, a large library had been destroyed; not a book that was not torn to pieces. It was not a cheerful walk.

Monday (November 28).
While waiting for an answer from Versailles, I must amuse myself; so, I walk about the town. The Mother took me to several hospitals, where I saw much suffering and very much dirt. They are twenty years behind us in all sanitary matters,—no ventilation, no proper food, dirty beds, men lying in their clothes, not even the floors swept. I'm disgusted.
We can hear the cannons distinctly, this is the third day. From one part of the city we can see two of the forts around Paris. Today I hear the French saying that the Germans are defeated; at any rate, the Sisters are quite gay over some news.

Tuesday (November 29).
Went this morning to see Count P. He has had no letter yet, but promised to come after twelve to see me. He and Dr. H. came together. Count P. was indignant that I had such quarters, and took me at once to a nice house on the hill. The garden is full

of flowers and I have a good fire. It is pleasant to be warm again. A good *Deutsch* Sister from a nearby hospital sends me my food; and now while waiting I would be really happy if I could have only one letter from home. I have written so many.

Wednesday (November 30).
I took a long walk in the country and had such a good time. I went to a village about two miles away. The people called out "Dutch, Dutch;" they saw the cross on my arm. Can anything in the world be dirtier than these French peasants? I have never yet seen a nice face; and when one sees the bent figures of both men and women, one can believe the French nation is decadent. How can such mothers bear heroes?

Thursday (December 1).
Last night the first wounded from the battlefield arrived, and this house is made an officers hospital. Among others was brought a colonel wounded in both knees and in the ankle. I have been up all night. The poor man is suffering more for his sons than for himself; he has two, both wounded, and he knows not where they are. The whole street was full of wounded men. I feel as if I were back again in our War; only here there seems no order at all; everybody flies about distracted. The way they dress wounds is abominable; they are not even where we were in '62. The surgeons have had a consultation over the colonel, and have decided that he is too old for amputation. In America, they would have decided differently, I am sure. So, they have put the worse wounded leg in a plaster of Paris bandage. God only knows how it will be.

Friday (December 2).
A whole deluge of Sisters have come from Stuttgart. They insist upon coming in and taking everything out of my hands. I stand my ground as well as I can; but they have the whip hand, for they can speak better than I. Anyhow I won't do servant's work! I'm an officer or nothing. I want to go farther forward at once; but Count P. will not let me stir until he has the long-waited-for answer from Versailles.
The colonel has revived so much. I have been to other hospitals today, and I can hardly contain myself to see the treatment of the wounds. It seems actual murder. We never treated amputations so badly;—head, hands without any care, and the men al-

lowed to eat all they will. I can see now how good our surgeons were. One good thing they have here is carbolic acid in all its forms; this alone will doubtless save many lives.

Saturday (December 3).
I can't get up the least enthusiasm. In the first place, I haven't enough to do, nor can I get it. I think there is one woman to every two wounded men,—all with caps or some such costume, and calling one another "Sister." Prince von Weimar was here today, and I asked him to send me forward; so, he gave me a letter of introduction; but Count P. says I cannot go yet. I'm pretty mad!

(Lagny), Sunday (December 4).
The day is not marked, as with us, by inspection, though, Lord knows, it is needed. I have come out of the hospitals to-day feeling just grieved to see how everything goes here. And there is no excuse, for the houses are large and supplied with every convenience, and there is an abundance of food; but it is cooked like Satan. I have not had a bed since the wounded came; but that would be nothing if I could eat once a good meal. I can drink the wine; but I don't like it, it's so sour.

(Lagny), Thursday (December 8).
The days are all about alike. I do what I can; but it's useless breaking my head against these time-worn customs. Thus far every amputation within my knowledge has died, excepting one; and if he doesn't he's a fool, for there is no reason why he should live. There has been no amputation in this hospital, I am glad to say; if there were, I would have to fight.

(Lagny), Friday (December 16?).
There has been a snowfall. Till now the gardens have been green, and with so many vines and flowers blooming; but this ends them. I've been out hunting for a washerwoman, and have found a little Frenchwoman who will do. She is the only decent-looking one I have seen, and she's no beauty.
It is some days since I wrote. I have since then left the hospital I was in, and have been for some days in the Pension Fleury, the vilest place for dirt and smell I have ever been in. The Sisters are Catholic, and so mad because I am here. I have seen a number of operations, and never have I seen anything so abominable.

One amputation occupied nearly an hour, and was performed by three surgeons who, in the end, were covered with blood. The patient of course died in four hours; why he did not die during the operation is a mystery. I was disgusted, and said so to Dr. D., who agreed with me, in words at least. I have determined to leave here anyway. If I cannot go forward, I will go back, and join the English ambulance at Épernay, or else go to Zwickau (her husband's birthplace).

I cannot get transportation any farther. This hateful Count P. has refused me even to Meaux, though I have a letter from Prince Weimar saying I shall go. Whether it is that I am not Catholic or that I am American, I do not know. I will not stay here much longer. There are crowds of Sisters here. Every cook and chambermaid in Germany who wants an adventure seems to have put on some peculiar cap (they wear no bonnets) and started out. Banded together by dozens, they fairly storm a hospital, and after a day or two all are driven out by them. I have not a bit of a chance because I do not speak quite fluently; and now I've had enough. I will see Dr. D., the chief, tomorrow, and get his permission to go back to Épernay.

My dear friend whom I nursed, Colonel ————, is dead after all. When tetanus appeared, they concluded to take off his leg. Dr. D. refused, knowing that, without the operation, he might live till his wife came, but that it was too late to hope for his recovery. But some wise man from Stuttgart came and said it must be done. They had only made the first cut around when he was dead. I am so sorry for his poor *frau*; she came next day, only to see his dead body. Poor wife, she has already lost one son in the same engagement, and the other lies hopelessly wounded an hour's ride from here. *La guerre!*

December 17 (?), Lagny.

I depart tomorrow, at five o'clock, for Épernay. I have been for some time quartered on a French *dame* who seems really sorry to have me go; but I leave here without a single regret. It is the forlornest place that can be thought of,—so dirty, so disorganised in every way, not a decent hospital in the town. What can be expected when all the wounds are dressed with raw cotton, carbol oil, flannel bandages, and oil silk, besides a heap of nasty lint? Not a single amputation of the leg, so far, has lived;

hardly one of the arm, and those are doing badly enough. Every wound, for a *finale*, is covered with a triangle of cotton; these triangles are a peculiar German institution and are used for everything. How I do long to have one wound in my own hands!

18th, Épernay.

I arrived here this morning and have seen the English Dr. Frank, who was so kind; but I have no chance here. He has a whole band of English Sisters, who, by the way, can't speak one word of German or French, and yet all goes good. It is the only hospital I have seen in the least approaching ours excepting Dr. Brigham's at Noisiel. Dr. Frank gave me quarters in his own house, and I passed such a delightful evening with him and Dr. Montgomery. I needed this little comfort, for I was quite discouraged. He gives me letters to the English ambulance at Metz; so, tomorrow I start again.

(19th.)

Rode all day and passed the night at F———, as it was too late to go to Metz. It was dark and rainy and so muddy, and I had a half hour's walk to my quarters."

There is no entry in the journal until March 30 of the following year. The rest of her wanderings towards the goal for which she had been always aiming, Vendôme, are partly chronicled in the following two letters, all that remain of the many which she must have written.

United States Consulate, Reims,

Friday, *le 23* December, 1870.

I do think this is the last time I shall have courage to write; I have come away back here expecting to find letters, and not one here; but the feeling that I must accomplish what I came for prevents me from returning. Not one word have I ever heard since I left New York; and yesterday someone told me that he did not believe a single letter of mine had ever left the office at Lagny. What will you think if you have not heard from me? I was so disgusted there I could not stay longer, and found it was impossible to ever get any farther; so, I determined to come back and join the English ambulance at Épernay. I arrived there Tuesday; but Dr. Frank, who is most lovely, had just imported a band of English Sisters, and so needed no more, as he has less than fifty beds and five or six Sisters; but he gave me letters to the English ambulance at Metz, so I went there. (By the journal the arrival at Épernay was on December 18, which was Sunday. There is a hopeless confusion of days and dates at this period.) There they have only French patients, all old wounds and *beyond* nasty. Such a place was never seen. We don't know anything of such things. I stayed there two days, but he (Dr. ———) has all French Sisters who won't work with anyone else, and he himself is an old fool. I'm sure he never saw a gunshot wound, or, indeed any. I have before described the dressing of wounds here; he's a little behind that even. Won't God punish such murderers! I have seen more suffering than ever in my whole life before. Our war was nothing to it.

(Later.) I am now writing in the cars, for I am on my way to Orléans with letters to English and American surgeons; somehow, I feel as if this was the turning-point in my adventures. I keep a journal of everything, so all you miss you will know when I get back. I will not write one word about my experience, for I know all letters are watched; but at least you will hear that I am alive and have been well ever since I came to Europe.

Orléans, January 6, 1871.

I am sure of this letter finding its way to you, and so I write with real good heart; one of the English surgeons goes home tomorrow, and has just told me that he will post it out of the war region.

I had a very hard journey from Épernay, (through which she passed in going from Reims to Orléans), I can assure you; and without the hope of getting to the English ambulance I would have given up many times. From Nanteuil to Meaux I came in a baggage car full to the brim with matter for the hospitals. We had to ride all night or, rather, make stops all night, as such trains always do; and it never was colder. My seat was a salt bag; could anything be worse? I thought I should freeze, sure. We had no light, and I did not know a soul. I shall never forget the length of that night. Such a Christmas morning! But the *commandant* at Meaux gave me quarters in a cloister, and they treated me well,—gave me a warm chamber and a nice dinner; so I soon got comfortable and then went to see Captain N., the English Chief of Ambulance there. He was real good, and, as the next morning he was sending stores to Orléans, promised me a place in one of the wagons.

Captain N. said we left at seven, so I had coffee and started before light; found, of course, nobody ready and the goods not loaded; so, it was a long wait till ten o'clock, when the three wagons started loaded so heavily and with all the drivers (English) drunk from too much Christmas. The two officers who conducted the expedition were very cross and didn't know the way, and it never was colder, so I have sometimes had a jollier ride.

We got only twenty-five miles that day to Brie, a little town where the famous cheese is made. I had quarters in a fine old house with two of the funniest little old women and a nephew just like them. They were evidently frightened out of their wits, and seemed to think I would eat at least one of them. They put one foot-stove (*chaufferette*) in my lap to warm my hands and one at my feet, and flew round like two very old hens; they ad mired everything I had on and myself generally. The house was so damp that I wondered how one could become so old in it.

We started rather earlier next morning, but nobody felt just right yet and we had various accidents through the day. When we got to Corbeil they refused to take the goods by rail (here the road commences), so we went on to Juvisy. This is the most remarkable town I have seen; it is full of *châteaux*, so old and fine. They said positively here that we could not go on by rail; they go only by horses, having no engine; so, we looked round for lodgings. That was not to be thought of,—five thousand soldiers there and it but a very small town.

So, after dusk, we started again; every moment seemed colder; and (give me an American for all the English in an emergency) "we ga'ed and we ga'ed" to find an old castle where they said we could have quarters. We rode at least ten miles round, and at nine o'clock we found it. A great, old, rambling place with huge halls and rooms that it was impossible to warm. A colonel was quartered there with his regiment; he was very cordial and gave me his room. We had a nice supper with him and some good wine; but the bed was so miserable and the house so full of noises that I could not sleep. I got up early in the morning and took a long walk through the grounds and garden, which are wonderful, sloping away down to the Seine and full of statuary and arbors, and so quaint and strange, with a most picturesque old church. The place was the Château of the Jesuits,—ever so old. The old fellows were turned out when the soldiers needed it.

It was late when we left, and then we found we were only one mile from Juvisy after our long ride; so stupid! We went back to Corbeil, and there I determined to go on. They left me and went back to Meaux; stupid things! they could just as well have gone on, for the next day I found a German party who have much more than they, and, by insisting, we got through. The first night we only got back to Juvisy; there everything was unloaded and it looked rather bad for us.

There were five of the party: two doctors and two gentlemen from Frankfort going for wounded friends to C.; they were decidedly the pleasantest people I have met all the way through, so jolly and yet so gentlemanly. We could not even get anything to eat, at first. Finally, one officer told us he would give us something to eat if we would find a place to cook it. He gave us coffee, canned beef, vegetables, and pork; so, with all our hands full we started to search the town. Finally, after a great run, we got a chance at a fire and two pots; and by and by we had a capital dinner.

Then we had to find lodging for the night; that was more difficult. At last we came to a great castle (this all sounds like *The Mysteries of Udolpho*) occupied by a regiment; at first the *commandant* said no; but when he found there was a lady (and it was so horrid cold and already dark), he said if we could sit up all night we might come in. I would willingly have consented to stand on my head, I was so tired and cold; so, he brought us through these elegant apartments into such a splendid room (or rather hall, for it was perfectly immense) filled with everything beautiful,—exquisite paintings and statues and such gorgeous furniture and books and music and an immense marble fireplace full of wood, which was best of all. We drew our chairs around the fire, drank red wine, and laughed and talked till at last we all fell asleep; and really it was a nice night. As to the whole castle I will tell you about it sometime; it was wonderful. Some of the Orléans family own it. I fear not much that is fine will remain when the soldiers leave it.

We were fortunate enough to get a pack wagon; so, we rode all day through the most lovely country and by such charming towns and *châteaux*. It was horrid cold, but I was bound to see everything. Our party was very jolly and we had plenty to eat, though it was frozen. We got to Étampes by dark; there we had to stay all night, and the crazy old engine brought us here next day. It always breaks down, but it was good to us. Here our party separated, much to our regret.

I have been quartered with a most charming old couple; he is one of Napoleon's old officers (I mean the first Napoleon), and is so full of interesting stories; his wife was a great *belle*. They remember all the revolutions, and I should be real happy here only I can't get into a hospital; they are sending all wounded away, and the Anglo-American ambulance will employ only Sisters of Charity, who won't work with anyone else. But Baron S. sends me tomorrow to Gien, where are many fresh wounded; there I hope to find a hospital.

I'm afraid to write one word of war news for fear my letter won't reach you; but today the news is not very favourable for the Prussians. They have, however, been bombarding Paris for some time, and at Juvisy, where we were so close to Paris, we could hear the firing night and day. There have been terrible battles the past three days on both sides of us. I hope to get my letter from Épernay. Oh, dear, I never expect you will; though as to myself, if I get much more discouraged, I shall go back. It's no use to ask you to find me; write to Berlin, *Poste restante*. I will find letters there, or perhaps may have a chance to send for them.

Chapter 9

At about this time Mrs. von Olnhausen seems to have put herself, or to have been placed, under the direction of the *Johannitern*, or Knights of St John, those modern representatives of the old Knights Hospitalers.

By this Order she was sent towards the front, by *diligence*, accompanied by a Knight of St. John and by two unfriendly Sisters. In this not wholly agreeable company, and worn out with the long buffeting from place to place, the homesick and emotional little woman was quite overcome, on the second day of this journey, to see waving from a beautiful *château* the American flag. This proved to be the Château de Meung, owned by an American but confiscated by the Duke of Mecklenburg for the use of the German Army.

Here Mrs. von Olnhausen remained two weeks, doing what she could for the patients there under the difficult circumstances of being almost totally ignored by her fellow-nurses. So, hostile were they that they did not even inform her of the retaking of Meung by the French, and made their preparations for a hasty departure quite without reference to her. Fortunately, the Knight in charge of the hospital was more friendly, and made the diligence in which the nurses were to be taken away wait until she too could make ready for departure.

This last removal brought her to Vendôme; and thereafter, under the direction of the medical staff of the army (between whom and the *Johannitern* there appears to have been much jealousy and friction) she was given the recognition and the work which she had so long sought. The *maire* of Vendôme, moreover, at whose house she was billeted, proved the best and most influential of friends, giving her cause for everlasting gratitude.

Arriving at Vendôme in the latter part of January, she stayed there until the 30th of March. As long as the German Army remained (it was withdrawn from Paris on March 3), the conditions were most comfortable and agreeable for her; but the general order for evacuation having been carried out, she was left for several weeks practically alone in the midst of a hostile population and in charge of critically wounded men.

This period, and the still more dangerous and wholly futile journey, with eight patients, away from Vendôme, is quite fully covered by the extracts from her letters and journal which follow. That experience was the last of the many disagreeable adventures met with in France. Arriving in Berlin, she was soon greeted by her late husband's sisters (who had heard of her presence in Europe only through the efforts of the officials to trace the owner of the missing trunk), and was taken by them to their home in Tharant, near Dresden.

Vendôme, February 16 (1871).

I have often had the excuse of feeling too sad to write; but I think never, until now, of feeling too happy. Yesterday, for the first time since I left America, I have received letters from home. I have tried to avoid telling you how unhappy I have been about it, and always have spoken hopefully when I have written; but now you must realise how much I have suffered. I am so glad I have had the courage to wait and not turn back, as I have so often been tempted to do. To be sure, the letters were all written last November; but I'm so grateful for that much. I have already written you about my life here, which every day I like better. I cannot say too much in praise of the first doctor that I had. He was nearly as good a surgeon as Dr. Bellangee; and the one I have now is excellent, too. Moreover, they have learned that they can trust me, and so they have practically nothing to do with the wounds.

They are evacuating here as fast as possible, and have already given up the school to the city; so, I have now a large, fine room in the old hospital. And I have the same good luck with the wounds that I had at home. I think, too, the men like me as well—perhaps better—than if I were a German. You would be surprised how well I can speak both French and German.

The church, as I wrote you, is very beautiful; and since I last wrote I have found time to go in. I have seen no such paintings in France in any church, and the old windows are most wonderful, though many of them were ruined when they blew up the bridges. I often go in now, and am quite friends with one of the priests, who wants always to ask so many questions about America. All the French seem to think that's the best land, and I'm treated with marvellous respect when they find that I am American.

I still like the Sisters very much. They are not imaginative damsels; but the older is well educated and plays nicely; which is pleasant when we have any time to spare. This, however, is not often, for it is frequently nine o'clock when we sit down to dinner. However, hard work makes good digestion, and I don't care how much I dream so that I dream of home.

I suppose if we really have peace one of the terms will be that the Germans shall leave France at once; so, we may all have to go. I shall be really sorry not to see Paris, and I shall try my best to get there. Aren't the conditions demanded by Prussia hard? And they are starving there in Paris while the world decides. Here we can already live much better. The people are bringing out their stores, and we don't get the everlasting answer: "*Rien du tout, du tout, du tout,*" no matter what we asked for.

I could always get more than the Sisters because I told them I was American; so off would come their hats, and, after searching in some horrid, dirty, old back place, they would bring something to light. Speaking of this, I say the French people are the dirtiest on the face of the earth. Their houses, especially those of the peasants, are abominations. You see, I poke into every house, under some pretext, and have thoroughly learned their "tricks and their manners."

The town is already full of people returning from their flight. The small-pox has been dreadful here, and so fatal. The bells are always tolling, and the priests forever singing in the streets with candle and cross, followed by such a motley crowd. They always go on foot, and it's no short walk to the cemetery. It's well they have something to do. The mayor told me there were more deaths here in the month of January than had ever occurred before in an entire year.

Right in front of the window where I sit the river runs, with only the street and a little garden between; already the spring birds are singing, and the air is soft; and the street is full of market people crying their different wares, with their white caps and blue linen clothes, so unlike anything one sees at home. The wonderful old clock in the town strikes the hours and quarters so musically, and the sun shines so brightly on the warm yellow stones, it makes one quite happy. It has already struck the hour for my going to the Hospice, but I still sit; and now that Sister Marie has brought me a strong cup of coffee (meaning the coffee), I feel wonderfully content. I just have seen a boy pull a fish from the river which I have a great appetite for. He looks very ragged and nasty (I mean the boy, of course), so when I have done I shall go out and lay hands on him (I mean the fish). A couple of *sous* will make both him and me happy.

Dr. Lazarine (?) , who has been here a week with the Sisters, has given us lots of good things. He goes back to England tomorrow, and I shall be sure then that this letter, which he takes, will reach you. He is such a kind old man. Not one of the doctors speaks one word of English. Oh, yes, one of them does. A young fellow says "All right," "Beautiful," and "My dear." Whenever anyone speaks to him in English he always makes one of these for answer,—he says he must keep up his English. He is bright, and I think one of the Sisters and he are quite in love; so perhaps she will not always be a Sister.

I told you in my last that I should go on to Meung; but now I shall not go. When my doctors found that the *Johannitern* wanted me to go there, they vetoed it at once, and said they would give me all the work I wanted. So, they sent away the men who were well enough and gave me all those who were really bad. There is such jealousy always between the *Johannitern* and the regular army. Since then I have heard that the English ambulance is there.

There is no other letter for a month, but it is clear that the interval was quietly spent in work at Vendôme, under fortunate conditions. Meanwhile the preliminaries of peace had been signed on February 26, the German Army had entered Paris on March 1, and the return to the Fatherland had begun.

Vendôme, Thursday, March 16, 1871.

I wrote a week ago that I should leave the next day (Thursday), but just as I was getting into the carriage the doctor sent me word it was impossible for me to go, as they had received eight very badly wounded men from another hospital and he wished me to have the care of them. I was delighted, first, at the compliment, and then because I wish so much to remain in France till warmer weather; it is so cold in Germany. I can't tell you about these men; I have never seen any so bad. They have had no care, have lain wet for weeks, and have such sores and such indescribable wounds. I am busy from early morning till nine at night.

I have left M. Sarazen (Mayor of Vendôme) and am now with my friends the Mesdemoiselles F., who are the loveliest, kindest, funniest old women I have ever seen. The moment I enter the house they dance around me as if I were a queen; and when I undress they stand admiring. All my clothes are folded like a child's, my shoes cleaned, my bed warmed, and a bottle of hot water placed at my feet; and in the morning they are at the bedside to see that all goes right; while in my dressing-room are a good fire and warm water. I'm sure they feel rather aggrieved that they can't bathe me. They are so puckered up, so very little, with grey hair so very much frizzled, and they talk so fast.

What one says the other always repeats. They are aristocrats of the old days, have seen terrible times, when their friends were dragged to the guillotine under their very windows. The brother, who is a facsimile of the sisters, comes to the hospital with me when it rains, and I find him at the door when I go out. Everybody calls me "Madam American." For the last two days, I have been indescribably happy, for I have had the first letter from home since those written in November.

This is such a pleasant old town. I believe I've seen everything that one can see except the old clock, which I am going to visit today. Now that they have no longer fear of the soldiers (who have all departed), the children are pretty saucy, and when I put my head in the street call out, *Prusse, Prusse*; so, it is better for me not to go alone anywhere.

Day after tomorrow the doctors and all the hospital corps depart. I alone remain; but you must not be worried about it. It is impossible to transport these men by wagon, and the French will not give us a train at present. I would not leave these wounded men, though the doctor-in-chief says I may go if I wish. I think the French will respect me more, as I am American, and I can interpret for the men, not one of whom can speak a word of French. You would be surprised to hear me jabbering French now, and German; I have no longer any need of an interpreter.

Sunday (March 19).

This has been such a dull day and so long, the patients are so sad. Four have died since yesterday morning. I feel tonight as if we should all die here together. I have now nine left, three wounded, four with typhoid, two with small-pox. I have everything to do, and it is vastly harder when the men are low-spirited and have so much to fear from the French. My doctor came to pay me a last visit on Friday evening and spoke so nicely of my staying here alone; in the morning when I saw them all passing before the house, I felt strongly tempted to go too.

★★★★★★

The following translation of a letter from this surgeon is of interest in this connection:—

Vailly Near Troyes, April 30, 1871.

Most Honoured Lady,—I have just received your letter, and although I have not read it because it is in English, which along with several other languages I do not understand, nevertheless, I will answer you circumstantially. Just as two soldiers who have fought side by side are bound for their entire lives by this brotherhood of arms, so you, most esteemed friend, have always been the faithful companion who sacrificed herself for the welfare of the wounded; and I have never found anyone who was more self-sacrificing in this service nor more reliable. I have often gratefully remembered your forgetfulness of self in this great calling, and have often reproached myself for having left you alone in Vendôme in spite of the fact that you desired to remain there. With due regard to those poor people who had to stay behind, we could not refuse your self-denying offer, and we were influenced, too, to accept since we were sure of your capable help, and I am convinced, although I have not yet read your esteemed letter, that you have fulfilled your task as conscientiously as successfully. I have often spoken of you and sympathised with you since you were left alone in Vendôme, so I am all the more glad now to receive not only this token of your esteem, but also the news of your safe arrival.

I am glad that you, at least, who have really earned it by your self-sacrifice, are in my dear Fatherland and with your people, while I am still far from my family—my poor wife and my four-year-old son. I am quite sad when I think of it, but when I consider the numberless widows and orphans who, comfortless, await our return, then I judge myself fortunate.

We had on our journey to Blois, then by rail over Orléans, Étampes, Juvisy, Corbeil, Melun, to endure many hardships; afterwards we marched by way of Nangis, Provins, Villenauxe, to Troyes. We have been encamped now for four weeks not far from the latter place (nine kilometres), and the end is not in sight. I shall endeavour to have your most friendly letter translated by a comrade. It will please me very much, however, if you have time, if you will write me a few lines in reply—in German or French, perhaps Polish, which I also understand—or to have that done. In case I find no one, who will translate your letter for me, I should be very glad if you would translate its contents briefly into German, which perhaps you will do anyway, even though I find someone to do it for me.

Farewell. I think of you with most grateful reverence, and of your good heart.

With many greetings, your friend and admirer,

Dr. Schwerke (?).

★★★★★★

Friday (March 24).

I have not found time to write one word since Sunday. I find the patients here so different from the soldiers at home. I have never known the names of one of them. They accept everything as their right, and are always so impatient and obstinate, and it is not the same pleasure to take care of them as in our war The news from Paris is every day worse, and I think the sooner we are off the better. This morning we had a telegram that we must leave tomorrow morning, but two are too sick to go. I hate to leave them, especially one who was amputated the day before the doctors left. The other it matters not, as he will die. The poor fellows do not know yet that they must stay, and I dread to tell them. I think they will die from fright. Did ever such a people live as these French! One would think they had enough with such a war; but now they must fight with each other. (The uprising of the *Commune* began on March 18.) The people are furious that the prisoners are still detained in Prussia.

The next letter, written from Berlin on the anniversary of the Battle of Lexington, gives quite fully the story of the eventful weeks following March 24.

> Berlin, Wednesday, April 19 (1871).
> I'm just glad enough to be back here, feeling that now I can hear regularly from you and you also from me. You can't know what a cross it has been to me, and nothing but my Yankee grit ever carried me through. I think if I had found nothing to do I never should have had the courage to go back to America, though now you may feel assured that while I had anything to do I worked with might and main; and you will be satisfied, I think, with what letters I have from my doctors.
> You will wonder where I have been all this time. I wrote last from Vendôme. I had all my men that could go ready, and when I found those that I could not take feeling so bad to be left alone, I decided to go only to Blois, and then to return and stay till they were better. Just as the wagons were prepared, however, came a despatch saying that I must wait a day or two; so, I put the men back in bed, and you may know that was a blue day with all. Now they thought they never would get back to the Fatherland. I began to think so, too; besides, I had so little money left, and, to keep them alive, I must buy them meat and wine at least.
> We waited a week, and it looked gloomy enough, when Thursday evening, March 30, just as I had finished my rounds, the mayor came in with a despatch from the *Sanitätscommission Agent* at Orléans that I must leave right off; so, at six I was at the hospital, and by eight we started. I forgot to say, though, that in the night another man died, so I had only eight to take with me. I rode in the *coupé* of the *diligence* with the two smallpox men, who were really better than they looked,—in fact, the only two who could sit up. It was market-day, and the town was full of people. The mayor was anxious on that account that we should leave early, as they are bad enough with the Prussians. Luckily, we got off without being seen by many; those who

saw us shouted and ran after us; but the drivers were real good, and we were soon out of their claws. For me the ride was especially delightful after my long confinement; but the men were so tired and so hungry and so cross!

When we got to Blois, we found we could not go on to Orléans; there was a despatch awaiting us that we must rest for three or four days. I was not sorry, for the men were used up, and Blois is full of interest; it has the most wonderful and best preserved *château* in France. Nothing was ready for us. They were breaking up the hospital, so we had to wait an hour in the wagons. Then the chamber was so cold, and the stove smoked, and the horrid stone floors, which we always find here, were so unbearable. As soon as possible I had them in bed and a good supper for them. The people were very kind and showed the greatest sympathy for me, so I too had a nice supper and a good enough bed; but as I had to watch and do everything, having no one with me, I could not rest much, for the men were too tired to sleep.

After I had made them all comfortable in the morning, I left my smallpox men for watchers and went to see the town and the *château*. I was gazing, bewildered with its marvellous beauty and interest, when up came a man with a despatch to the effect that we had twenty minutes to get to the station. Such work! I had all the men to dress and prepare, while somebody got a carriage and men to carry the stretchers. "Batterman," the newly amputated man, I took in the carriage with me; the others were on stretchers. I had only one blanket to cover him, as I had to send the others all back to Vendôme; but I supposed, of course, that there was a *Sanitäts* train for us.

When I got there, I found nothing but a pack-wagon, and no straw, no mattress, not a thing; and this man only fifteen days amputated! Even what little time I had was used up in quarrelling with the Inspector of the Station. He said positively I could not go; there was no requisition for me, and unless I paid full fare I must stay. I felt amazingly like breaking down; but I brought all my French eloquence to bear, told him I was the same as an officer in charge of those men, and go I must; so, at last he brought me a paper to sign stating I was an officer *pro tem*, in charge of eight Prussian soldiers. Wasn't it most lucky, for I had spent my last cent that morning? When all was done, he said I had still ten minutes. The men were lying in the *salon*; those who had come on stretchers had their own blankets; but they had taken Batterman's blanket to lay him on, and there he lay with nothing over him. I had no time to get anything for him; even my waterproof was in the baggage car; so, I took off my dress and skirt to cover him and rode to Orléans without. I had to sit on that dirty floor and hold his head, and was nearly jammed to death, to say nothing of the cold, for it was raining hard. We were more than three hours getting there; I thought it ten.

When we arrived no one was there to receive us; what could I do? I thought every moment two of the men would die. Some-one brought the inspector, whom I shall always remember with real affection. He was so good (though a Frenchman), sent at once for a mattress and blanket, had the men put in the salon and a fire made, and then sent for the *Sanitätscommission Agent*, whom he knew. After an hour that official came, with a very red nose, and so fussy and so frightened that he did nothing but turn round. I was disgusted with him. He insisted upon speaking English, and the devil could not understand him. My German is perfect in comparison.

He said he had everything prepared at the hospital, but how to get there was the question. I made many suggestions, which were put aside. After an hour's talk, he decided on what I had at first proposed: that the three wounded should go on stretch-ers, the others with me in an omnibus. Then a stretcher and six men had to be hunted up (think of the condition of the sick all this time). At last all was ready, when the inspector said we could not go without *gens d'armes*; so, we hired two. Mr. S. C. Agent then concluded he had something else to do; but I think he was afraid to go. Anyway, he let me set off alone.

The Prussians had left Orléans three weeks before, and the peo-ple supposed all had gone. When, therefore, they saw us, they hooted and screamed, and one horrible old woman howled out all sorts of curses, kicked up the dust over us with her awful old wooden shoes, and shook her head so that her grey hair fell over her face and shoulders. I never saw such a fiendish face. I could then understand what a revolution in France meant. The men were dreadfully frightened; but we got to the hospital safely, and I felt glad enough.

I expected to stay there all night, but the Mother said no stranger was permitted to stay in the building unless sick. I was rather in despair; but I borrowed some money from one of the men, and passed the night in the most miserable of little inns, the master of which boasted, while I was eating supper, that he had been a *franctireur* for three months. All the company looked so too; but it was Hobson's choice with me. As I was to be at the station at six, and must rise early enough to have the men ready, I must be as near as possible to the hospital.

I went immediately to bed, but such a room! I feared I should oversleep, so had told the man to call me at five, sure. I thought I heard him knock and sprang up; hearing the clock strike at the same time, I hurried on my clothes and opened the window to listen for the carriage and the man who had promised to be there at half-past five. I got so impatient as the quarters kept striking and nobody came; at last the clock struck *one*. I was too mad, and so cold. I would not undress again, so passed the night in that miserable, half-awake state till half-past five.

When I rang at the hospital gate, I found the men nearly ready, and that the Sisters had given them some bread; then I looked again for the carriage and my *gens d'armes*. Finally, they came, but not my stretcher-men; so, I flew about the street begging everybody I met to come. Finally, I picked up six of the lousiest, lost-looking wretches ever were seen, and started for the station, the same crowd following and "a-cussing."

About ten minutes after I got there Mr. S. C. Agent arrived with twenty other men that had been forwarded from little stations around; they had all had small-pox and looked rather shabby. He himself flew round like a parched pea. "What had we better do?" was always the question, when there was only one thing *to* be done,—to get the men in a pack-wagon speedily as possible, with plenty of straw, which he ought to have had ready. Thanks to my friend the inspector, this was accomplished, and the men were covered as well as possible with all available coats and blankets, when the bell rang. I had got only six of my men and one other in my car when in rushed the agent: "Madam, here is a despatch saying all must wait for the ambulance train, which comes at nine o'clock." I saw nothing else to do but wait. "Yes," he said, "*you* must do so, but I think I'll go as far as Juvisy and wait for you there; it's so dangerous here!"

So, my men were taken out again on the platform, and there I was left without one *sou*, one friend. Again, my inspector came to me, put my men again in the saloon, lent me five *francs* to buy them a breakfast, and locked the doors to keep out the crowd. Nine and ten came, but no train; every five minutes the men would say, "Oh, Sister, won't you go out and see if they are not here?"

Ever since I have been left alone with them I have been Sister Anne to them, always looking out to see if help was near. When twelve o'clock came and no cars, and the men got hungry and weary beyond endurance, I went out for the last time, determined to go to the mayor and have them taken back to the hospital; when, behold, "the cloud of dust," and directly the doctors were with us. We all cried a little, and now there was no more delay; the men were soon warmly in bed and fed, and I had quarters with the two Sisters (Protestant) who always go with the train. I found them very dirty, but very hospitable; any way it was so good to have this terrible anxiety over, that I was content with anything.

Now commenced our journey. We went to Tours, where, by the way, I met some delightful Americans: Mr. Lee, from Baltimore, and his wife, from Rhode Island; they were very nice to me, and I spent such a pleasant afternoon with them. They have done so much all through the war for both sides; they live there while educating their children. From Tours (which is, by the way, a beautiful and rich city and less destroyed by the soldiers than any other, for which they have to thank Mr. Lee, who persuaded General Hauptmann not to quarter his soldiers on the people, but in the *casernes*) we went back to Vendôme. Wasn't it abominable in this S. C. Agent to make me take all that horrible journey for nothing just because he was afraid himself to wait any longer and dared not leave us behind?

From there we have been journeying ever since, through such a beautiful land. It's three weeks tomorrow since I left Vendôme the first time. We have stopped at nearly all the large cities through which we have passed long enough to see the best part of them; at least long enough to give one a desire to see them again. I especially enjoyed Ulm, Munich, and Nuremberg; in each we passed a day or more. In one we were two days, so I made good use of the time. I have kept a journal of all my journey. I know such things are horribly stupid, or I would send it to you.

Although this journal to which she refers covers very much the ground of this letter of April 19, it is by no means "horribly stupid," and it differs sufficiently from the letter to make it worthwhile to reproduce it, even though the facts are mainly those already given.

(FROM THE *JOURNAL*.)

Blois, March 30, 1871.

We left Vendôme at nine this morning, my two worst wounded in one wagon, the other six with me. All the rest are dead; the last died last night. I was glad when he died, for I could not have brought him, and I hated to leave him in France. The day has been beautiful, and the ride altogether lovely. We found nothing ready for the men, so had a half-hour to wait before I could have them in bed. The chamber was cold, and the floor, as always in France, of stone. We are in the wonderfully beautiful *Château de Blois*, the most beautiful in France.

My men were so tired and hungry, I fear they will not sleep well. I have a bed in the next room; I dare not leave them, and, besides, I have no one with me to do anything for them. I am very tired, and am glad to hear that we must stay here for two or three days to give the men rest. The people seem kind and have given the men a good supper. As I look up at the old walls, I cannot realise that I am here alone. How did I ever dare to come as I did, not speaking the language and not knowing one person in France? I could not have come if I had known how hard it was to be. Now that I can speak it is different.

Orléans, Saturday, April 1.

This morning I had so much to do, as I have no one to help me except the hussar who has the smallpox. The men were tired and out of sorts,—I have never seen them so impatient. After they were cared for, I went into the town with the hussar to buy wine and bread. The people followed us in crowds, and some of them spoke so meanly. But I always answer good-naturedly, and it generally ends in a laugh. But it certainly is not pleasant to be alone in *Frankreich*. I am always anxious for my men (not for myself), for the French nature is so uncertain one can never know what may happen.

After I came back I gave the men their dinner and had a good one myself. The Sisters here (Franciscans) are very kind, and seem delighted to talk with an American. Then I went to visit the *Château de Blois*.

I can find no words to tell how wonderfully beautiful it is. I did not stay half long enough, for in the midst came a man with a despatch saying that we must leave Blois in twenty minutes. My Lord! I had all my men to dress and make ready for the journey to the station. They sent Batterman in a carriage, but the others went on stretchers.

When I got to the station, I found no ambulance train there, and, while I had requisitions for my eight men, I had none for myself. So, I had a very stormy time with the inspector of the rail road. He said positively I could not go. I said positively that I would, that I was an *Officier Américain* left in charge of the men to conduct them to Berlin, to which place they and I would be transported. Until the last moment he held out. Then he brought me a paper to sign, as is required of all officers, and let me go.

All this time my men had been lying on the floor of the waiting-room. They had taken Batterman's blanket to carry him in, so he lay there with nothing over him. I demanded a pack-wagon to carry them in, as they could not sit; so, they were put in one. As Batterman had nothing under him but his blanket and nothing at all over him, I had to take off my dress to make him warm, and I thought he would die before we got to Orléans. It is not yet three weeks since his leg was amputated, and it is marvellous that he survived that ride. I cannot tell how I pitied that man. I had to hold his head all the way, and was myself cold enough when we reached here.

There was no one in waiting for us, and I did not know what to do; but the inspector was very good, and had the men taken into the waiting- room. He then sent for the agent, who ought to have been on the spot. It was an hour before he came, and then with so much cognac in the head that he was little better than no one. Besides, he is so afraid. I never saw a man so frightened. It was a full hour before he got together the men to carry the stretchers, and a carriage for me. Then we must have *gens d'armes* to accompany us, as it is not safe here without them. It was rather a mournful procession to the hospital, and such a gloomy place when we got there. The men were all tired out and were glad to get to bed. The hospital is the *Hôtel Dieu*, in charge of the Dominican Sisters, who dress in white, and from the time they enter the house till they die never step out of it.

The old Mother—who is cross enough—would not let me stay there; so, though it was dark, I had to hunt up a lodging for the night, as we are to leave for Juvisy at five tomorrow morning. As I have not much money, I could not be fastidious, so am in a miserable little inn in which the people all look like robbers, with most villainous faces. They set before me a scanty supper which I had no appetite or heart to eat.

Orléans, Sunday, April 2 (1871).

This *is* a day. I'm sure I shall never forget it. It began altogether wrong, for I thought I heard the knock on the door which I had ordered the woman to give to waken me. As the clock was striking, too, I leaped out of bed and dressed in a hurry. Then I went to the window, which is opposite the hospital gate, to wait for the carriage and the men who promised to be there at five. After waiting till the clock struck again, I discovered it was only *one*, and that I had been dreaming instead of really hearing the knock. I was too mad. So, to bed I went again, almost frozen and with boots and clothes on, altogether so miserable. Of course, I slept no more, and felt as though I were a hundred years old. Finally, I got admitted to the hospital, made my men ready, and then waited so impatiently. When it was nearly six, I took a man and we went to hunt up somebody to help. Finding somebody at last, we reached the station just in time to put the men in the pack-wagon. This time there was plenty of straw, and I thought we were to be quite comfortable.

I had seated myself on my box for a little rest, when the agent (the same man I saw yesterday and who has managed the whole concern) rushed up and handed me a despatch to the effect that the ambulance train would be here at nine, and that I must wait for it. So we had just time to get the men again on the platform, when the train went off. I begged the Agent to stay and help me; but he said he had all his things in the car, and that he did not like, anyway, to stay longer in France. So, the miserable man went off, leaving me with those terribly sick, tired, and hungry men, and with not one cent of money, and with no one to help me except the hussar. I have never been so near despair; but I had no time for that. I hunted up the inspector, who was kind and had the men put into the *salle*; and here I must wait with them for the train to come. They had had no breakfast, and I was too sorry for them. Again, I had to apply to the Inspector, who lent me some money to buy them a breakfast.

At last nine o'clock came, but no train,—so ten and eleven. I was at my wits end. The eight men were all crying with pain and cold, the room was full of French soldiers and "blue blouses," who were so hateful, and, if the train should not come, what could I do? When at last I saw three doctors at the door, I could not keep the tears down. They were so nice, and had the men put into the cars at once and fed. There are two Sisters (Protestant) on the cars who have lived thus for five months. They have given me a bed in their car, so I am right comfortable. After dinner, we went into the town. The people are bad enough, and it would take very little to make them wicked. We leave here at ten tonight for Tours.

Tours, April 3, Monday.

We arrived here at five this morning. We find two wounded men here, but there are many in the little towns around; so, we must wait here some days until all are brought in.

April 4, Tours.

I was so disappointed this morning. The doctor went to Meung and promised to take me with him; but, after all, left me, for some reason. Someone told me there was an American family here, by the name of Lee, who had done so much in the war; so, I got their address, called, and was so delighted with them. They were most cordial, and I stayed the greater part of the day with them. It was so good to hear American news. She told me so much about the war that I had not known before. After I left I took a walk around the town.

(Tours), April 5, Wednesday.

This morning I took a walk to the *Château de Beau Jardin*, which has been used for a hospital, but which I was not permitted to enter. I am the only one that dares to leave the cars, and everyone thinks me rash; but I find the people very polite and kind. Somehow, I always find such pleasant people wherever I go. The doctor has returned this evening with ten sick and wounded men. We leave at ten o'clock tonight for Vendôme. I have no patience when I think how badly this thing has been managed. I could have had my men so comfortable all the while in the hospital instead of taking that hard journey, had it not been for that stupid Agent. It is a shame to give such a man such a place. He was sent here to hunt up the wounded, and he has left without giving the doctor any information at all,—just frightened out of his wits.

April 6, Thursday, Vendôme.

This morning finds us at Vendôme. A week ago, tomorrow we left here, and now we are back. It seems a month. I had such a horrid, anxious time. I must go to my friends the first thing; so, as soon as we had seen the doctor, to learn how long we are to remain here, we (the two Sisters who travel with the train and myself) went to the ruins and to the cathedral,—which is well worth seeing,—and then to the F.'s. (See mention earlier). They were so cordial and glad to see me, and insisted that I should stop with them; but that I could not do, as we may leave at any moment. We await only a despatch from St. Calais.

It was well that I did not stay in the town; for the doctor sent for me at nine o'clock to ask if I were willing to go to St. Calais for him. The surgeon-in-chief had gone to Blois, he (the doctor) could not leave, and I was the only one who could speak French. I was delighted, of course. Besides, I can go where I will without fear, as all in the town know me, and I have only to declare myself an American to find friends everywhere. So early in the morning I shall go into the town to find a carriage and start for St. Calais.

April 7, Good Friday,

I have passed such a pleasant day. It is a beautiful drive to St. Calais, and the little town is a charming place, lying under the hills, so white and clean, and with a curious old church in the Roman style, with quaint carvings and statues. There is a ruin, too, very old. I had time, while the horses rested, to see all. I then started back with my one poor fellow who had been so long lying in the hospital here alone. At first, he did not want to come. He felt safe in the hospital, and thought, when he got out, the people would be so bad to him. But after we started he was very glad, and arrived here not so much tired as I expected he would be. It was quite dark when we arrived, and, as we leave in the morning, I shall not have time to say *adieu* to my dear friends here.

April 8, Saturday, Corbeil.

All the day we have had the most charming drive through such a lovely land. As we near Paris, it becomes every moment more beautiful. We left Vendôme very early, stopped at *Château* ——, found two men there, and stopped for an hour at ——. The country is here very beautiful, the fruit-trees all in blossom, and everywhere such splendid *châteaux*. Wherever we stop the people flock to see the cars,—the first ambulance train they have ever seen. Everywhere we heard such bad news from Paris. In one place, near Juvisy, we saw from the cars a long artillery train coming from one point to attack the city in another. The most demoralized soldiers (not even excepting the Southerners after the war was over) that I have ever seen are these Frenchmen,—

dirty, ragged, haggard, miserable-looking fellows. I cannot conceive how the army ever had the prestige that it had. Such women and men as one sees in the fields cannot bear heroes. Juvisy looked bright and pleasant. It is a lovely town; and I saw the two castles where I passed those two nights here. I'm glad it's not so cold now as then. There are still Prussian soldiers here. It seemed very good to see them again.

(Épernay?), April 9, Easter Sunday.

We stayed at Corbeil till the afternoon. I took a long walk, and heard Mass in the old church. I never saw such stupid girls as these Sisters. They are content to stay in the cars and never see one thing. It was just so with the two Sisters in Vendôme; all the time we were there they saw nothing, and yet were never half so much with their men as I was. We used to walk, and I must always say "Look there," or they would see nothing. "Born blind." It's my third visit here, so I feel quite at home. We ride as far as Sans tonight.

Chaumont, April 10, Monday.

We arrived here at noon and stayed all the rest of the day. I was so provoked that I did not see the town, which is very lovely; but they told me we might go at any moment, as we were only waiting for a despatch. Nothing is so dreary as waiting at a railroad station. The day, too, has been so beautiful.

(Nancy), April 11, Tuesday.

We left Chaumont only this morning. The ride has been very nice today, especially the last part, as we neared Nancy. The crops are all in, and the grain looks miserable. I don't see what the people will do another year for food. We arrived at Nancy sometime in the night.

April 12, Wednesday, Nancy.

All the day long I have been in the city,—in the morning with one Sister, in the afternoon with the other,—so I am thoroughly tired tonight. I saw only my friend the German Sister at the convent *De la bonne Chrétienne*. The person I most wished to see, von Havernich, is not here. I shall never forget that man's kindness to me (presumably while seeking her lost trunk) when I was here a stranger. He had gone to Metz for the day.

April 13, Thursday.

We left Nancy and have travelled all day through Lorraine. Immediately one can see that he is in another land. The German element is very perceptible, the houses and villages are so different. The people

162

mostly speak German, too.

April 15, Munich, Saturday.

It is delightful to be here, it's such an interesting city. I intended, after breakfast, to go alone into the city, but it rained hard. Besides, the doctor sent word that all must stay in, as the queen comes. I have not the slightest desire to see her; but one must obey orders. (*Later.*) The queen has been here; but I did not see her. The Sisters are quite enthusiastic over her amiability, etc. It still rains. I'm disappointed, for Gustav has told me so much of Munich, I want to see it all.

April 16, Sunday, Munich.

We are entertained by the Sanitary Commission, so we have everything good to eat and drink; and after breakfast the gentlemen took us for a drive past the university and to see the statue of Bavaria. That alone is worth coming here to see. The temple is beautiful, too, in the court of which it stands, and is filled with busts of illustrious men. It looks out on the immense plain where the October festival is held, so vast, so green, and the whole city lying beyond. From there we went to the cemetery, filled with beautiful works of art, but all crowded and jumbled together.

The saddest sight I have ever seen is the dead house, where all the dead must lie three days in full dress with wreaths and flowers, uncoffined for all the world to see, before they can be buried. I think there were twenty there, some children of only a day or so, and some people so very old. We leave tonight at nine for Nuremberg, where we stay a day.

Nurnberg, April 17, Monday.

This is the most marvellous old town I have ever seen. Every house is a study, the people are so friendly, and the streets are so crooked and steep and queer. We went first to the churches, and then to the fortress and museum, where are kept all the horrible instruments of torture. I cannot realise that so late as 1863 a man was here tortured, with his wife, for stealing. They were put into a large cradle filled with iron spikes, and there rocked for some hours. The woman died, I'm glad to say; but the man lived and was afterwards imprisoned for eight years. Here were the wheels and ladders, racks, iron whips, iron masks,—I cannot remember all the horrible things I saw. We went then to a beer house four hundred years old to drink beer and eat sausage and *sauerkraut.*

Fulda, April 18, Tuesday.

The ride has been very fine today among the mountains, their high points crowned with old castles and ruins, the little villages with their red roofs looking so cosy, the people, when we stop, so friendly. We stopped for a while at Neuhof, and I was so struck with the people as they came from the little church. Everyone had a bright handkerchief tied on the head, a large woollen scarf crossed on the breast and tied behind, and a strip of velvet around the skirt, the colours being of every conceivable shade. The effect was beautiful. They had such sympathy for the sick men and for us who cared for them. One woman tried to give me two little pieces of money. I could not take them, but the act touched my heart with such a glow. I wish now I had taken one as a memento. She looked very poor, and told me that she had lost her only son in the war. Fulda seems to be a fine and rich city, but we cannot see it. We leave all our sick here; I do not know why. Only two or three go to Berlin with us.

April 19, Berlin, Wednesday.

We arrived here at noon today. I hurried for letters, but found only one, of January, from J. It's so strange, and has quite dampened the spirits I was in at getting here. I have to comfort myself writing to them and also to Madame von Roemer (her sister-in-law).

164

Chapter 10

Arriving in Tharant in April, 1871, Mrs. von Olnhausen shared the life of her husband's sisters and other relatives for more than two years. As will appear, this visit was interspersed with journeys to Berlin, to the family-seat at Zwickau, to Prague, and, in the spring of 1873, to Italy and France. This longer journey was taken in the capacity of companion to a widow whose nervous invalidism made the care of her an exacting and not altogether pleasant task. Glad as Mrs. Olnhausen was to get this wider view of Europe, she was not a little relieved when the time for ending this temporary companionship came, and she could return to what was now a home to her in Saxony. The von Olnhausen relatives were most cordial and devoted, and urged her to remain with them indefinitely; but their brother's wife was too sturdy an American, was too deeply attached to Massachusetts and to Lexington, to permit of her staying abroad longer than until the fall of 1873.

The letters from Germany are very voluminous and are practically intact. But the greater part of their contents is of too personal and intimate a character for publication. Sufficient extracts will be given, however, to present the extraordinary juxtaposition of a perfectly unconventional American and her strictly conventional German sisters-in- law, brought up in the atmosphere of generations of *Freiherr* tradition. Their brother's widow was an unending surprise and shock to them. She was as scornful of German usage as of the intricacies of German grammar. To her the elaborate etiquette of the German upper class was as superfluous as the cases and genders of the elaborate German tongue; and she usually flouted both.

To her the limitations placed upon the actions of their women were as absurd as the variations in their conjugations; and she took a free-born American's delight in ignoring the one and the other. But her unconventionality, and her love and practice of liberty, could not conceal, even from the eyes of German tradition, the nobility of her nature, the fundamental good-breeding of the real gentlewoman. And, however she might scorn local and extraneous usages, she was too true a woman ever to go counter to essential courtesies. Therefore, not simply as the widow of their dearly loved brother, but for herself, those fine old German aristocrats took her to their hearts, and took her also—of course with apologies for America,—but never with apologies for her into that exclusive society which the average American can see only from outside. The following letters, shorn as they must be of personalities, can give but an inadequate picture of that life which, in their entirety, they set forth so well. Those previous to June 15 are too personal to be given.

Tharant, June 15, 1871.

The paper you sent is the only American paper I have read since I left America. How long ago that seems! Do send me the other one you spoke of, if you can find a copy. I wish to see myself in print. As to the story of the Irishman's leg, I've forgotten about it; did I really cut it off?

I told you in my last about J. (Frau von Roemer); she perfectly worships Gustav's memory, and is good as pie to me because he loved me. I think, as she and L. (Frau von Rohrscheidt) say, they would carry me on their hands when they could. L.'s husband was a colonel, who died a little more than a year ago; he had six children when he married her, and they had three; but all of them love her so much. One is a colonel, one a major, two were captains, and have left the service.

Of these one has a rich wife and immense estates, the other married a noblewoman in every sense of the word; she had no money, though, so he is a coal-merchant; and all the family, except the mother, are so indignant when they see the wagons go by with von Rohrscheidt on them. He says he is much prouder of that title than if he were idle and were called count, and he means, too, that his children shall be so proud of it that they will add it to their coat-of-arms.

You ask me how I look. I'm not so horrid fat now, though I am by no means wasted; but my clothes feel more comfortable, and, when my hair is dressed, for an old lady who must wear glasses I look pretty spranky. J. is so interested, as is L., in all of you. She remembers everything Gustav ever wrote about you all, and I think reads his letters over every week. The dear Uncle K. is dead; when he heard of Gustav's death, he said he wanted to live no longer. He placed all his letters on the table, and always had them there till he died; read them over and over, and often said he had nothing more to live for now his dear son was dead, for he always had felt Gustav was his son. I have seen Uncle K.'s sister, a proud old lady, in Dresden; she kissed me, held me long in her arms, and said I was a happy woman to be loved by such a man. She is such a wonderful specimen of an old-fashioned lady,—so straight, so well and richly dressed, and so ceremonious; I guess she never forgets herself. She is eighty-five, is such a little thing, and steps around like a princess. She seemed to me just like some fairy godmother who could turn us all into gold and silver if she would.

I shall pass a day with her soon. Before I finish my letter, I must say a little about the German fighting. I agree that they are good fighters, but not that they are the best soldiers in the world. I have had a chance to see both wars, and I'm sure I don't boast in saying that the Americans were the better of the two. We had a much worse enemy to contend with. What had the Germans? A people who at first didn't want to fight, hated their leaders and emperor, never had one good general, were perfectly unprepared and undisciplined, were badly clothed and fed from the first, and felt their inferiority.

The leaders had no faith in the men, and the men no faith in the officers. Two of the best fought battles were lost by the disobedience of the soldiers, who would have fires though strictly forbidden. There was no sentiment on either side, as with us, and the Germans had only to go right along and take, or buy, everything. I like the Germans well enough, Lord knows; but I want to see them fight with a real nation before I quite yield the palm to them. When I think of all we had to contend with, I think again that that was the War of the world.

Tharant, July 13, 1871.

Although I fully enjoy European life, when the time comes to go home, I shall be ready to enjoy more than ever our own land. I feel every day more proud that I am an American. Only by going to America can one get out of the narrow circle that binds one down here, especially in the life of the aristocrats. I guess the *burghers* know how to have a better time; the fear of what people will say is not so great with them. For my part, I don't care. I won't do anything unladylike,—or what I think is so,—but if I choose to go through the street of this little town without gloves or in a calico morning-dress early in the day, I do it; moreover, I speak to people, even if they have *not* a half-dozen titles. As to saying all the polite things that one must say here, that's entirely too tiresome.

I came back (from Dresden) the 3rd of July; it was the first morning of the return of the soldiers, and I found the town beautifully decorated with triumphal arches, and with garlands and wreaths hung from every house. As the soldiers marched through, the ladies, all dressed in the Saxon colours (white and green) and looking very charming, threw bouquets, and gave them beer and bread and butter. The castle of Count Zokorisky (have I told you about him?) was hung with garlands and flags and looked splendid. Even the old ruins were decorated.

The first regiment, the crown prince's favourite, was quartered here. All the officers are noblemen, and the people were, consequently, delighted to have them. The sisters would not have officers, so had each two or three soldiers, who were fed and cared for like children. It seemed as if L. could not do enough for them,—besides beer and all sorts of things for dinner, they must have a bottle of wine and cigars, and she was always cooking for them.

I believe every day but one the city has given a concert, sometimes ending with a dance. We go at three with our work (the German women would die without their knitting), and talk over coffee, being always joined by some acquaintances. Not the least amusing part is watching the people. When we have been at home, we have had many visitors; for L.'s husband was formerly in the same regiment, and all the older officers were friends. Twice we were serenaded, too; so, with the continual repairs necessary to bring my shabby wardrobe up to the required elegance, you can see I had really not a moment to write. For the Grand Review, I received a ticket to go with all those who nursed in the war. The Tribune was especially for us; we all wore our Sanitary scarf with the red cross, and there was not a better place to see in all the city. I went in from here (to Dresden) at six in the morning, took coffee with the S.'s, and then drove in their carriage to see the decorations of the city, which were the finest I ever saw. This took two hours, and we came back for breakfast at eleven. Then we went to the Tribune, which was rather killing, it was so hot, and it was twelve before the procession began.

First came the king, a little, old, bent-up man in uniform, looking not at all kingly; then the queen, who looks good, with her daughter and grand-daughter, the crown princess and Princess George, who every one said was handsome, but not one of whom looked so to me. I was so mad, too, that they didn't have crowns on their heads and sceptres in their hands, with spangled garments, as we always see them painted. I know if I were a queen, I'd *be* one.

Processions are always alike, I suppose, but really this did not seem half so fine as some I've seen at home. I was quite disappointed in it. I think, in the first place, the soldiers don't compare with ours, and there was so little enthusiasm with both the soldiers and the people. I remember the review day (of the troops returned from the Civil War) in Boston when every step was a heartfelt ovation.

At nine in the evening we went out to see the illuminations, which weren't very good, after all; and then came a thunder-gust and blew them all out and sent us scampering home.

I am not even allowed to dress my hair; everything is done for me as if I were a child,—and such people! I suppose these *grandees* would be shocked to know I had ever stood at a wash-tub three days at a time. I, too, begin to forget all about it, and already am very much like the young damsel who forgot what a rake was.

(Written to a child)

Tharant, July 26, 1871.

I must first of all tell you about the Children's Festival (*Kinderfest*) yesterday, which was so beautiful. Ever so many years ago somebody died and left money to the city for giving every year, in July, a festival to the children (that was a good man, I'm sure, and for that deed he must have gone straight to heaven); so, every July that comes. Rich and poor all unite on that day. There were hundreds there; all the children must have a wreath, and, however poor the mother is, she will have a white, or pretty calico, dress for the children. Even the babies in the wagons had wreaths on. In the morning at five o'clock the drum beats all through the town to waken them. They are all washed and dressed neatly, but not in their best (that comes later), and all meet in the market-place, where they form a procession and march with music and singing to the school garden, where a tree is planted. They go all through the town with banners (I forgot to say that the teacher makes in the garden an address, the preacher a prayer, and they sing a hymn, all very short, but nice). The sheriff goes before with two other officials, and orders everybody out of the road.

After this they all go home for rest till three o'clock, and then come together, old and young, in a large garden here with a wonderful lawn, and there they dance and play all sorts of plays, and sing and have a feast,—a very simple one, beer and a kind of buns, and bread and butter. Every year they make a subscription among the people and have a lottery; the teachers give each child a ticket, and everyone has a prize; and it's so nice to see the bright faces. They all go home in the twilight as far as the market-place with music and banners; there the teachers say *adieu*, and all the little white darlings scamper home with their treasures. It was so pretty, and everybody had such a good time. The children here have such a pretty fashion; after they have eaten, they go all around the table and kiss the hands, and to the father and mother they say, "I thank you for my dinner," or whatever meal it is (*ich danke für mein Essen*); isn't it nice? Another pretty thing is, the youngest one at the table always is called upon to ask the blessing. It was so lovely the other day; some friends were here with a little girl of four years; she folded her little white hands and spoke so reverently; it was beautiful. This is a queer, quaint old town altogether; a stream about ten feet wide runs through the middle of it; on each side is the street; of course, it's very crooked because it follows the stream. Then everybody has put his house just where he wanted it; so, there are all sorts of angles, now wide, now narrow. Nearly close behind the houses rise the mountains, so most of the gardens are terraced up; the stream is crossed by little foot-bridges, very shaky and badly railed; so, every now and then somebody tumbles in, and is taken out with broken bones. This week a lady died who fell in one dark night; but still nothing is done about it.

Sister L. has the most wonderful hens for laying I have ever seen; I don't know what breed they are; some are speckled and some black. She always keeps ten and a cockerel (I'm sure I don't know how to spell that word); and from the first of March till today they have laid seven hundred and eighty eggs. Sister has a regular hen-book, which is kept with such care; all she buys for them and all they do. She is very methodical in everything; indeed, I think all the people are much more so than by us. Everything is kept under lock; the sugar-bowl (or rather box) is always locked, and the tea too. All the drawers and closets, and even the comb and brush box, are locked; for my life, I can't get used to this custom, and they are always running after me with my keys, which I'm sure to leave in the lock.

Sister gives her maid twenty *thalers* a year and her living, and how she does have to work! Ours would think they must die with it all. Nobody has carpets; so, all the floors have to be scrubbed, great brass door handles and locks must shine every day, brass pots and pans for cooking in numerable glisten like gold, every morning the windows must all be wiped and very often washed. Moreover, there are the hens to feed, the garden to tend, all the ironing to do, and most of the washing, the stone stairs of the house from top to bottom to whitewash once or twice a week, all the errands to do, besides all the ordinary house work, which is not light. What would Miss Biddy say to this? And all without a murmur. The servant women save money, and some time will marry and be able to buy a cow and pig, and perhaps a dog and wagon to carry their milk to market.

Sterne, near Prague, August 19, 1871.

I tried to write you before I left Tharant, but it seemed impossible, for we would make the house very fine for the mother when she comes home. You see these *Deutchers* (*sic*) would go on for hundreds of years and never move a chair or table from its original place; but I saw at once so much that could be bettered. I took advantage of L.'s absence and whisked everything about. M. (Fraülein von Rohrscheidt) at first looked on in surprise; but pretty soon the same spirit came over her, and, *whit*, the whole aspect of the house was changed. We sawed down uncomfortable tables and chairs, took off doors and hung curtains in their place, and hung the mirrors so that people could see their elegance in them. I knew if I did not do all this myself, M. would never dare, and I'm sure L. will be pleased because I have done it; she is quite foolish about me.

The entrance to Prague is most beautiful, especially through the *Baumgarten*, which is the pleasure-ground; and the view of the city with its hundred towers and its splendid castles can't be described.

We got up ever so early, for the children (L. has four) wanted to see the wonderful (great-) aunt from America, and there was no sleeping after they were awake. The moment we had coffee the children were made ready, and we all came out here with our work into this immense garden,—"King's Garden;" and here we have sat all day long. Look where you will are groups of people sitting at tables or on the grass, eating, drinking beer, knitting, or sewing. Hand-organs are grinding, and everybody, when a drum is played, joins in the wild dance,—mothers with their children, maids with their little boys and girls; it's too pretty.

This is a favourite summer place, with the most abominable holes to sleep in; but nobody stays a moment indoors. After they have had coffee, all take dinner and supper here. Living is so cheap in this land; there were today three of us grown people and four children, and our whole dinner—beer and all—cost not quite fifty cents; and we had a right good one,—*Schnitzel* (veal cooked in some good way); *Dampfnudeln* (I'll send you the receipt for them); beef with ale sauce (which is real good), and beer.

That I don't drink, so I had a glass of white wine; but you should see the Bohemians once drink—no, not drink; they open their mouths and let it run down,—men, women, and children. There has been no rain here for some weeks, and the leaves are falling from drought. The wells are kept locked, and all the washing water must be bought and brought up the steep hill on the backs of these poor, overworked women in a kind of wooden tub, which is so heavy. It makes my heart ache to see how the poor must work here, especially the women.

All the children here—the babies, I mean—are wrapped up to the arms in a feather or down pillow, which is bound around and around with bright ribbon. Think of it, and the thermometer at ninety; and when they go in the wagon they are covered with a down cover besides. I want to fight with every mother over this; but they all say the babies would die without it.

Goodnight; I hope you will sleep better than I know I shall, with the windows closed and with four children, a maid, and three grown people in two little rooms; it is worse than the prairie.

Tharant, September 9, 1871.

Monday, I took my last turn around the city (Prague) and felt quite mournful that I should not see it again. I wanted especially to visit the old Jew quarter once more. With all its filth and smells, it is most interesting. One is carried back so far on seeing that old church which was built in five or six hundred. One feels really dumb in such a place.

I went once more to the Hradschin, the palace of the kings for many centuries. I wanted to see the hungry tower that no one else cared to visit, they think it's so horrible. On the first floor are the cells where the state prisoners are confined for life. Those are bad enough; but below them is where those who were to die from hunger were placed. Around the central hall are the smallest kind of cells, where men were chained to an immense beam running across a grated window.

Here they must listen unceasingly to the cries of those chained in the circular hall to a stone bench running around the chamber. In the middle of this chamber is a round hole, which is the entrance to another very deep cell, into which men were lowered by a rope. One by one they were let down into this hole to die of hunger, and those above must hear the howls and ravings of these wretches, unable to help them, and knowing it to be their fate also to die in the same way. Men lived generally eight or nine days in the hunger cell, and then the bodies were thrown into a still deeper hole, and the stench from that made it even more dreadful. I have no patience when one talks of the "good old times."

I felt as if the dust of ages had settled on me when I came out of Prague, all is so quaint and "old-timey" here. Of all the places where one can live cheaply, too, it is the first. For a half-*thaler* a day one is luxurious. The wine is delicious and too cheap, and the grapes are displayed in piles; one can eat all he will for two *kreutzers.*

When we got back here, the whole house was hung with garlands and wreaths, the loveliest tea- table was set out with flowers, and such a nice supper was ready. The Sisters were here to welcome us.

L. is the dearest soul in the world, but she has lived in the narrowest circle, and is constantly afraid of running against some old-time custom. For instance, no lady was ever known to drive here. Day before yesterday a Frau von K. offered us her horse and carriage, but only three could go in it; so, I said I'd drive, and then we all three could go. L. was horrified, said that had never been known in the annals of Dutchland; and it took all my persuasive powers to coax her to go. Now she must explain to everyone that American ladies are so independent, and that the richest and most elegant all do so there. It's so absurd. I hope I shan't do anything to disgrace my nationality, but I feel strongly tempted sometimes to do something outrageous. Now the ice is broken, I shall have many good rides about this beautiful country, for Sister was overjoyed at my not landing her in a ditch, and will gladly go again.

Tharant, November 20, 1871.
We went to a grand tea-party one night last week. First place, as soon as we came in, tea seasoned with vanilla was handed round, with cake and *Zweiback*, a kind of rusk. Then cards, talk, and a little music; and at nine supper, including five kinds of sausage (*Wurst*), herring salad, Russian salad, sour "*gouegous*" (pickles done like *Sauerkraut*), roast veal cold, roast mutton, coffee, two or three kinds of cake, wine, grapes, and pears, cold chicken, jelly, and, last of all, *Sandtorte*, the most horrible old cake made out of potato meal, that everybody thinks is too nice; it's just like sand. After this more cards, music, and talk; consequently, a very wakeful night and a fit of indigestion next day.

Tharant, Sunday, November, 1871.
Once a week we all meet and sew for some poor children, and on Tuesdays is the *Erholung*, when all the aristocrats meet in a hall. Till tea, we have reading, singing, or theatricals, and after that the old folks retire to the walls, and the young ones dance till nearly morning. These have only just commenced, and promise to be quite nice,—but the ceremony! At the last

one there were seven earls, and I don't know how many barons, most of them being students in the Forest Academy, besides so many from the town! This would give some of our people who come abroad talk for a lifetime. "My friend the Earl,—etc." Somehow, I'm not a bit impressed with the imposing situation. I see nobody more elegant and truly aristocratic than I know at home, who are only Mr. and Mrs.; but I really do enjoy seeing the life here, and I have come to be very critical, though I keep my thoughts to myself.

On the twelfth is to be the great ball of the year, where I expect to be overwhelmed with the greatness of the occasion. It's the king's birthday. I'm so mad; I'm considered too old to dance! Of course, I really am, but I do like to so much. However, the next best thing is to get beside some other pleasant old lady or man and laugh over all one sees. It's rather the fashion to talk with me just now, as I'm the first American woman who has ever been here in society, and it is rather refreshing, I guess, to see something or somebody new. I think I ought to go about with a striped dress, and with a liberty cap on my head, for everywhere I go I am known only as "The American;" the children all call me "*Tante Amerika*;" and as I'm always presented as "my sister from America," I'm more often addressed as "*Frau Amerika*" than by any other name. In France, I was always called "*Madame Amérique*," so I have to mind my P's and Q's that I do nothing to discredit my dear land.

Tharant, February 1, 1872.

I feel sorry that I have not written for so long; but, you see, when a fellow goes every night to a party or ball, and all the day has to make ball-plunder between the gaps, how can he write? I never dreamed I could come to such a life; truly, for the last twelve days we have not been a single night at home. I'm at my wits ends what I shall wear. I have turned and twisted my whole wardrobe many times; for one can't wear the same thing twice, and the fortune that is spent in decorations! I think every family has given or will give a ball, besides the *Erholung* and theatricals and coffee. I have been invited to two private balls in Dresden, besides, where were the crown prince and Prince George, with their wives; but I had to decline; it would cost more than I possess to buy *toilettes* for them.

I wish somebody who really liked great people had my chance. I'm sure they'd come home quite set up with their titled friends. I suppose I'm too old to appreciate such things; anyway, I don't find I have any taste for the great world. I am sure, though, if I were young and handsome I should be entirely spoiled; for everywhere I go I receive so much attention. But I'm more contented to sit in a corner and see all, and have something to tell you about when I come home.

Sister is in the city; she is full of business these days, as she gives a great dinner on my birthday (Saturday). All the family are invited, and she has been cooking for it the entire week; the house is scoured from top to bottom, fresh curtains are everywhere, and garlands and flowers. Such a fuss! You would think it was the queen's instead of my birthday; and when I think of the contrast, I don't believe it is I who write it. We are to dine in the big room upstairs, and all the best china and glass is already there.

If J. doesn't come and take me, I shall go to Russia to tend the wounded, if the talked-of war with England comes off,—unless we have the predicted war with Spain, when, of course, I shall immediately find the place where I am needed. My last experience in France has given me many new ideas with regard to the treatment of wounds; my long rest and good feeding have given me strength to go through a great deal; and my idleness has made me long for something really earnest to do. I feel like a wild horse with the bit in the mouth. Of course, I don't dare speak with the sisters about all this; they can't even hear of my going anywhere. J. is too funny; she is just such a lover as Gustav was, and I never open my mouth to speak that she does not fix her eyes on me. She often says, "Yes, Marie, I know now how Gustav loved you." The sisters all have said so much about me that it makes the people here most attentive to me. Everywhere I go, you'd think the queen had come. Then, too, I suppose my hodgepodge language is amusing.

Tharant, February 3, 1872.

I am just as happy as I can be this evening, and you too will be for me when I tell you that I have at last what I have so long wished for,—a *gold watch*. This has been such a pleasant day. The morning was beautiful, as the 3rd of February always is. Sister and M. came to me very early with such heartfelt wishes, and I found a birthday cake and many flowers when I went to breakfast. Then came my little maid, Minna Batch, with a wreath and a picture of a ship, and the best wishes written in a very crabbed little hand by herself. The others all came together, and all brought me flowers. The dinner was splendid. Many toasts were drunk. We drank many times to you all at home; then, after dinner, coffee and a good quiet talk together; and so, we sat till nine, when they went home. I've had telegrams and letters from all the relations, and feel quite set up with the fuss they have made over me.

Tharant, May 16, 1872.

This has been such a long, dreary time. I did not tell you why I wrote so little, for I would not make you anxious; but Sister L. has been so sick we have not hoped she could ever be well. I found it was better that one of us took the house; so, of course, I did. I've had a regular siege of cooking and general housework, for our one maid is generally running errands. There are, in a German house, five regular meals to get: the morning coffee and rolls, the nine-o'clock breakfast, the twelve-o'clock dinner, coffee and cake at three, and the *Vesperbrod*,—consequently much dish washing and cooking, besides providing for the outside company coming at unreasonable times.

At night, moreover, coffee and something to eat for the watchers. I've done it all with real good will, for no one else could, since M. has not left her mother for a moment. She was so sick, and such doctors! The first is the family doctor,—not so bad when one is not much sick. We all wanted another doctor, however, so he said we must have the one he usually consulted with. I wonder if any of you are old enough to remember an old doctor that used to come to see Grandma Phinney? I can't recall his name; but he was uncommon fat, had great warts on his nose, stuffed it forever with snuff, coughed and wheezed, and had his pockets full of herbs and things that smell so bitter and nasty.

Well, this second doctor was just his twin cherry. He came and thumped and punched a little, and said it was rheumatism, with a high degree of cold. We must sweat it out; so, he ordered that she be wrapped from head to toe in tow smoked with *Wick-*

rauch (vetch-smoke?), if you know what that is. I only know it smells good, and is used as incense in Catholic churches. Think what that poor soul endured for eighteen hours; even the hands were packed. At the end of that time she lost all patience and hope, and said she would willingly die, but she would not suffer that a moment longer. We, too, were past all patience, and finally telegraphed to the son in Dresden to bring out a new-school doctor. He came with a good one, who examined Sister thoroughly; and from that time, with his treatment, she began to mend. (She survived, however, only about two months.)

Tharant, August 19, 1872.

Our ride home (from Prague) was too pleasant; such a nice day, but we had one adventure. Mr. C. (an American) must rush out at Bodenbach for a cigar. Waiting for his change made him late, so he jumped on after the starting of the cars, which is a high crime here. Of course, the people called out; some said, "Jump off," and others, "Hang on tight." He, not understanding, was quite cool, and was making his way towards me, when it whistled down-brakes. The cars stopped and he walked in. Then you should have heard the storm,—the conductors all talking together, and the inspector furious. Mr. C. sat cool, and it only made them madder. I told them he could not understand, that he was an American, and "sich like." They said they did not care what he was; but when I appealed to their mercy, saying that I was alone there, they consented to let him go on, and we thought it was all over.

On arriving at Dresden, however, the door was thrown open, the inspector of the Dresden Station rushed in and said Mr. C. must come with him, as a telegram that he must be punished had been received, and marched him off. Of course, a big crowd collected, and everybody *hollered*, and nobody stopped to hear, till I got the floor and told them how it all happened; that, as he spoke only English, all was lost on him. "I'll make him hear," the official roared, and called for some other inspector who could speak English. The man came, and after much conversation they finally condescended to forgive him, with particular injunctions never to do so again. He said very meekly *he wouldn't!* and the disappointed crowd dispersed.

Tharant, October 24, 1872.

The ride to Neumark is so nice, and I saw for the first time Schönfels (birthplace of Herr von Olnhausen), which is on the route. You can think how I felt on seeing it. The two old castles can be seen far and wide; and, what is more, I was not one bit disappointed in them. After we got home (to Zwickau) we sat long in the twilight, and talked of ghosts and old times, till one began to feel cold chills over the back, as if ghosts of frozen mice were walking around; and the old pictures looked even more hideous than by daylight. It was proposed to go up to the garrets and hunt for spectres.

Someone said we must have a lantern, and just as I remarked, "No ghosts, of course, bring their own lanterns," the door opened slowly and one stalked in. You will not believe how we were all startled to see this immensely tall, white woman floating in with a lantern nearly a yard high and half as large round, a very ghost of a lantern. We all started up, for we had not missed Arthur, who had quietly stepped out, and, remembering these old things stored away, had improvised the whole scene.

Monday morning at nine S. sent the carriage to take us to Schönfels. It's about an hour's ride from Zwickau. We had many wreaths for the dead there, so first of all we went to the pastor's to get the key to the tomb. Here it seemed like some old dream; the loveliest little woman, so young and fresh and bright, came out of the kitchen and said she was the wife and would call her man. Soon he came down from his study, a *beau ideal* of a German preacher, so intellectual and so simple in manner.

The house was a picture of neatness and comfort. She brought us wine and cakes, and invited us to come and dine with them; but we had our own dinner with us, and we wanted that day to dine alone in the castle. The pastor went with us to the church yard and opened the vault, which was hung with garlands for one of the old Hempels who left a sum of money with which to give the children a feast every year. So, each year the children walk in procession, carrying wreaths and garlands, the vault is opened, and every tomb is decorated. This isn't an Olnhausen tomb; they are all buried in Württemberg.

Then we went to see the old church, which, by the way, was so injured by the earthquake last March that the tower had to be taken down and the whole rebuilt. It's full of interesting old monuments and slabs, flags and battle relics. After this we started on our pilgrimage, first, of course, to New Schönfels.

I don't believe a pilgrim to Jerusalem or Mecca ever felt more deeply than I did on nearing the long-talked-of home of Gustav. The owner knew J., and gave us permission to go all over the place. The house is inhabited only at night, the old man and woman going there to sleep; so, we were undisturbed. Everything remains nearly as when the Olnhausens sold it. The man has grown poorer every day, so nothing has been done to improve it; the old stag horns still hang in the hall,—such horns as one never sees now,—and stuffed birds shot by hands long dead are still ranged around. The same old papers on the walls and the immense wardrobes of polished oak, some of them so beautifully carved.

Gustav seemed to be by my side all the time. How often he has described it all to me! The old nut-trees that he loved so much are all dead; but the clock-tower is just as it was, and the old clock still rings out the hours to the village below. It must have been splendid in old times. The immense hall, on entering, and the broad old stairway are so fine, and there is *such* a view from the windows. We wandered about the park for a couple of hours, and on our return the old lady had a cup of coffee, and such bread and butter for us as I have not tasted in Germany. Her husband is most anxious to sell the place. When we came away, he brought me down one of the stuffed hawks as a remembrance from the old place (another trap!).

Then we went to the other castle, the von Roemers'. This is much higher and much older, and remains just as it was built. It is round, enclosing a court with very few windows on the outside, an old tower rising from the centre, balconies all around from the first storey, and such a gloomy aspect inside,—just the tower and walls with the irregular windows. The old stairs leading to the chapel are so neglected, covered with the same stones, old bones, and clumps of grass, bits of broken glass, and spider-webs that have been there for hundreds of years. There is one large hall where the whole Roemer family must meet once a year to hold council over the gains and what shall be done with them. The senior of the family has a right to live here, but hardly anyone in his senses would do so. J. was married here, and, as she is the senior's widow, has a right to live here always. She tried it for some years, but finally gave up her right.

They have lately dug up an old member who had long disappeared. He was a watchmaker (? manufacturer of watches), and has lived long in England. He finally announced his existence, and as it is a law in the family that they must pass some time of the year in Saxony or be not recognised any longer, he came and fitted up a few rooms splendidly, and has been here three months, and goes now back to Berlin.

We sent up our names and he gave us permission to enter. Everybody has much curiosity about him, he lives so entirely alone; so, we were most anxious to see the old lion and his den. He came forward very politely, and we tried our best to make him hear. He put his hand up and said, "I'm a little deaf." No adder was ever deafer. I bawled my best and, though he spoke English, which I tried at last, he only stared the harder at me and said "What?" in such an unearthly tone it took my wits all away. So, I left him to J., who managed to bring it into his head what she wanted.

He got the key, finally, and was a fit warder for such an old rumple of a castle,—a little, thin, dirty, brown old man with a very brown wig and white bristly hair cropping out, and such a wheezing and shaky tone; and such a suspicious look as he cast upon us every now and then,—on me particularly, as I wasn't a Roemer and couldn't make him hear. I wanted to go into the cellars, which are very deep and large, but Sister has not the taste for such things, and nobody in the castle has ever been there; so, I was obliged to come away unsatisfied. All around the wall is the old moat, of course long empty. Indeed, I can't see where they ever found water to fill it.

Outside is such a delightful walk on the banks looking out far as one can see, the other castle, the church, and the village all beneath you, and on hills away off other old castles. It was a splendid view, and enough in itself to pay for the clamber up the hills; but everything is so neglected and dirty,—even the village looks more like a Bohemian than a German one. By the time we came down the hill I felt a thousand years old, and the day seemed endless. As we went along, the people came out from every house and greeted the *gnädige frau*.

A. took us to Neumark, much to my chagrin, where we took tea with the family and then rode late into town, bewildered, tired, and actually bewitched, so that all night I could not tell if

I were waking or sleeping. Tuesday S. sent the carriage to take us to breakfast, and then she, the sisters, and I took a most delightful walk to the world-famous swan lake. Perhaps you've all read the fairy story of the swan Knight; here is the very place where it all happened. (The story of Lohengrin? The arms of Zwickau are quartered with swans and castles, and the name of the city is—erroneously—said to be derived from *cygnus*.) I am going to translate and send it to you if you haven't. It's so pretty, and is about as long as Walden Pond (Thoreau's *Walden*). Many swans are there, and gay little boats, and a big restaurant, and pretty paths all about; it is the pride and glory of Zwickau.

Tharant, December 8, 1872.
I write with ashes of humility on my head to think of my being hateful so long, and I have so many things to write about too. I never expected, after the week I spent in Dresden (which was the golden wedding one—of the King and Queen of Saxony), that I should wait so long to tell about it. The Thursday of that week was the christening of A.'s child, to which, of course, we were invited,—M. to stand godmother and I to help eat. There were six in the christening party. M.'s partner was a jolly man, Herr von W., who did not know how to hold the baby, and was withal so ashamed to do it; for, you see, everybody who stands up has to take the infant by turns.

The table around which they stood was trimmed love-lily with flowers, and there stood upon it a fine bouquet and the water. The minister, in robes, spoke for more than half an hour, giving a full history of baptism and its consequences,—which was drier than dust,—besides a prayer or two. Then the maid held the baby while the six people held a lace veil over it, upon which the pastor sprinkled water as he named it. Then he took the child, crossed and blessed it, and the thing was done.

They had a splendid supper and nice wine, and, last of all, the ice with a stork upon it. The belief is that whoever makes the stork fall will have the next baby. It fell to a young and very diffident doctor, who did not get over blushing all the evening. The young people danced and had a real gay time till two o'clock. I was sleepy enough to want to go home then, but the others stayed later and had another supper.

Next morning, we went to see the decorations, which, on the

whole, were tasteless enough, only that so many flags flying are always beautiful. The streets were crowded, with fine equipages rolling about. The people from out of Dresden were having audiences and bringing in the presents, so we saw much fine dressing; and fleas and noise were abundant. We were tired enough by two o'clock, and glad to get home. We had a good dinner and rest till evening, when we took another turn to see the illumination. This, after all, was not much, for the real sight was reserved till the emperor should come.

Every window had busts of the queen and king; in one of them the wreaths had got pushed out of place, and it had such a funny effect. This old lady with her nightcap on (for it looked just so, though I suppose it really was of superb lace), with one eye covered, looked uncommonly drunk, and he looked so rowdy I laughed and remarked upon it. This frightened L. so. "For God's sake, don't; if the police hear you, it will bring trouble;" whereat I shut up, having a holy horror of policemen.

The next morning, we stayed at home, reserving our strength for after dinner, when we were to go to see the emperor arrive. We got splendid places despite the immense crowd. We had many invitations to go to houses of our friends, but I preferred being on the street, so we went over to the *Neu Stadt,* on the square. The first thing I did was to make friends with a policeman, who gave us a front place and kept everyone from coming before us. There were some officers near who knew everybody and named them to us as they came along. We were so close, as they all passed in open carriages, that we could have shaken hands, and we got special bows; but I cared most to see our Saxon king, who is a noble old man, so good and wise. He has the saddest, sweetest expression. You know he is very learned in all sciences and is still a great student.

Sunday, we were early in the street. This was the wedding day, and oh, the crowds! You see the streets are so narrow all about the *schloss* that it seems much larger (the crowd, I mean); and such a hateful crowd, too, knocking and pushing. I was glad to find a corner where I could see a little. At last I told them I should go into the church. They all said it was impossible; but who ever knew a Yankee who didn't do the impossible? So, I screwed round to the back of the church, where the men go in, and pushed slowly along through the crowd till I got a good sight of the king and queen. Just then it began to rain, the people rushed in, and with a great surge I was pushed forward, unable even to move my feet, directly to the line held by the soldiers right in front of the whole party. Here I could see every one of them so nicely,—the king and queen kneeling together in one window, the empress alone in another, and all the other dignitaries.

A group of officers stood near, and one of them told me who they all were. Wasn't this my usual extra luck? But, oh, that music! If they have such music in heaven, one ought to want to go straight there. One would think the firing of the cannons and ringing of the bells would spoil it all, but it only made it all the more wonderful. I always shall rejoice that I was permitted to hear it. The king and queen both looked so sorrowful. After an hour, they went away; but the crowd didn't, as High Mass was celebrated; and I was glad I had to stay, for the whole music was so splendid.

(*Immediately after the golden wedding followed a short visit to Berlin.*) Monday morning, we went to more sight-seeing, and after dinner I called on Dr. R., who was not at home, to my disappointment. From there I went over to the hospital where my men were left when I came back to Berlin. At first, though I told them the date and some of the names, they were quite indifferent, and said they doubted if they could find them, it was so far back. Old lazy things! Besides, it was after visiting hours. Thereupon a young man who was sitting there rose and said: "I know the names, Herr Inspector; this generous lady nursed us all in that terrible time in Vendôme. I was one of them."

I was so pleased and surprised, and, as he stood on two legs and was so tall and fine looking, of course could not recognise him; but he told me (with some look of sorrow that I had forgotten him) that he was one of my amputated men, and had come back that same day to have his wooden leg better fitted. Of course, I had only seen him bolstered up in bed, very pale and sick. Then everybody flew round most politely, and an older officer, the head of the hospital, came out and took my hand, thanking me for what I had done. Very soon I had the list of every man made out. Only one was dead,—the one wounded in the thigh; the others had long been at home. The officer told me they had often enough spoken of me, and said some other things very pleasant to hear. My Pole, too, said goodbye with tears in his eyes, so I had a very comfortable ride home.

Mentone, France, February 7, 1873.

About four we left (Milan) for Genoa. You cannot conceive of anything more forlorn than the route,—just like our marshes, only the ditches are planted with willows. It began to rain, too, and a German gentleman gave me just at dark the delightful information that about nine we would come to a place where a tunnel was broken through, and where we must all get out and take ourselves for a two hours ride over the mountains.

I wish I could describe this getting out in a pouring rain, every step over one's boots in mud, men and women screaming in every tongue, pulling you and knocking you, cursing every moment, barely escaping being run over by such miserable beasts, too, and finally being thrust into an omnibus with five others in pitch darkness with a pair of horses that had evidently been trained to go on only two legs at once, the snapping of whips and shouting of drivers and jolting of the carriage into holes that seemed deep enough to swallow us, lighted up now and then by the glare of a torch or a great linen lantern (really coarse linen stretched over an iron frame with a candle inside), soldiers staggering along, for we had a regiment with us and they must all walk the whole route.

Oh, dear! I know you can't conceive of it all, and I'm sure I can't tell it. They say it is a splendid route by day, the view from the hills is so fine; but at night I would rather refuse to try it twice. Some of the carriages came to grief, but ours stood the test, and finally there was another struggle and howling till we were again seated in the cars, and were glad sometime in the night to arrive at Genoa, so "dead beat" that I could have slept anywhere.

As I left next morning (Friday) at eight, I had no chance to see the town at all, except the beautiful sea; and how welcome it was to me after hungering and thirsting so long for a sight of it. Nobody seemed to have any very definite ideas of the route; some said it was just impassable, some said we could not come through to Nice in two days; but I determined to try. There have been bad storms, and the road has been injured much. Of course, like all Italian roads, it's about half built; but it was not so very bad. Two or three times we had to get out and walk over

185

the worst places, and we poked along slowly; but we arrived at Nice at ten, having had the pleasure of having our trunks searched at the frontier town.

I drove to the *Hôtel Luxembourg*, where I found Mrs. C. expecting and waiting for me. I was glad to have the first interview over before I went to bed; for I dreaded it, not knowing what sort of a "critter" I should find her to be. To my delight she was nice and cordial, and seemed so glad to see me that I was entirely contented.

Rome, March 23, 1873.

I never saw such solemn people as in Rome. No New England town can beat it, for there at least you see contentment; but here extreme discontent, only the beggars looking bright when they have finally, with much screaming and running after, succeeded in forcing a coin from you. But you don't get rid of them as you hoped even then; for they still run and keep up the din, hoping to fool you twice. A Miss J. that I know here is very funny; she said after a while she would give only to the grey-haired ones; and then, she believed, every beggar in Rome put on a grey wig. Then she would give only to the babies; and every man, woman, and child appeared with one. A. says she will give only to the blind, but it seems as if everyone was blind; and even her good heart was shaken when she had no more coppers, and the blind man, opening his eyes, began to curse her.

While in Italy, Mrs. von Olnhausen received the Iron Cross. (The Order of the Iron Cross was established by Frederick William of Prussia in 1813. It was revived by King William, January 19, 1870.) This, like the Victorian Cross, is given for high bravery or special acts of noble service, and has been but sparingly presented. It is believed that Miss Clara Barton is the only other American woman who has received it. Accompanying the Cross was the following letter:—

Imperial Prussian Embassy.

Dresden, February 15, 1873.

Since His Imperial and Royal Majesty has deigned to confer by means of a supreme order of the sixth of January of this year upon your ladyship the Cross of Service for women and maidens, I have the honour, in obedience to an order of the Imperial Chancellor, to send to you hereby the Insignia in question and also a document for the Constitution of the Order, with the most obedient request to let the latter be returned to me after the separate rubrics of the same have been filled out.

May your ladyship receive the assurance of my sincere respect.

The Royal Prussian Chargé d'Affaires,

(Signature.)

To Her Ladyship
The widow Mrs. Von Olnhausen, per Tharand.

Later she received a war-medal (of silver) for non-combatants, together with a certificate for her services; and earlier she seems to have been presented with a medal of a more general character. After her return to America, a decoration still more rarely given, described as a Cross of Merit, was forwarded to her, but never reached her. At the time of Prince Henry's visit this was called to his attention by some friend of hers; and it was promised that another cross would be sent to her. Her death so soon followed that the promise, even had it been remembered, could not have been redeemed.

Tharant, May, 1873.

I must tell you about the wedding. Have you ever heard of *Polterabend?* The night before the wedding everybody who will give presents is expected to come and personate some character, or deliver an original poem, or do something to make fun for the others when he presents his gift. Generally, too, they dance till morning. All day long the relatives from a distance were arriving,—all sorts of big folks, with much gold lace and decorations on the men, and fine old lace and diamonds on the women. It was a hateful thing to me to have to be introduced to such a crowd. We went at six, still bright light and everybody gowned stunningly. Nobody else had the Iron Cross, so I felt more dressed than they.

For an hour or two it was the hardest work I ever did to get anyone to talk; but after the tea (delightfully flavoured with vanilla!) came in, we began to get more cheerful. In fact, I guess they were all hungry and cold, for it had rained all day. Then the chairs were arranged as for *tableaux*, and the presents were brought in. Some of the girls came in peasant costumes of their district, and had got some clever person to write verses, which were delivered in a half-scared, stumbling way, but which still sounded very good. One came as a flower-girl, brought a foot-stove covered with flowers, and spoke some very neat verses particularly well. Then came two for esters, classmates of Ro-emer, with big sacks on their backs and axes in hand. They had a long address, which was pinned up on the wall just outside the door, and first one and then the other took up the discourse as one or the other lost his place.

It was very funny, each one striving to get near the writing and never once looking at the bridal pair. They are both full of wit, graceful, and handsome. One had in his sack a splendid card-press, with counters and all sorts of things elegantly carved from wood, with the Roemer crest above all; the other had a beer-jug and glasses of white and green Bohemian crystal, and a waiter for them of carved wood with the arms at either side. One young forester came as a fox, and made such a nice, foxy speech. He ambled in and out so queerly, and pulled the string of his mouth with his paw when he talked, and insisted upon shaking hands at parting. His present was a dozen silver-topped corks, representing all sorts of animals and birds, on a silver stand, with a corkscrew of silver.

At nine we had supper, and then everyone seemed contented and glad. Roast veal, tongue, ham, salad, ice, and various half-sweet Dutch things that I don't usually gorge myself on, and a big bowl of punch which made everybody very merry. I must not forget one of the old *Polterabend* customs. All the outside friends come and dash against the door all sorts of crockery; such a smashing as one hears all the time! The more beloved one is, the more is smashed. Everybody saves up his old broken ware for such occasions. We could hardly get out when we would go home.

We left in a pouring rain, and woke up in the morning to find it still pouring. It was too bad, for the church stands so high and has no road to it. The hour was to be twelve, and we were all to walk in procession the whole way from the house with bare heads. The bridal veil did not come; it was promised the night before, but, of course, failed; so, they waited and waited. The bells began to ring, but the pastor was notified that he must wait awhile. At last a woman with a dog-cart came flying along with the veil, and the toilet was made. Then the bridegroom was not ready. In the meantime came messages from the bell-ringers saying they were worn out, as was the parson too. At the foot of the hill it rained like sixty, and we had to rush into the school for shelter, much to the disturbance of the scholars. There we had an eternity to wait, till finally we began the ascent between the drops. The little girls were to strew flowers, but they quite forgot to do it, they were so taken up with their fine dresses.

The church was crowded and as cold as a cellar, and everybody had a red nose and wet feet. The parson discoursed a full hour, mostly upon the greatness of the old Roemer house and upon its honours; and was too stupid for anything. Then the same rain to go back in as far as where we could take the carriages. The dinner was at the hotel at the end of the town. Over fifty guests were at table, and there was a constant ringing of glasses and wandering about drinking toasts. So, it was rather a confused time, and some of the dresses were quite ruined. After the hearty part of the dinner was over, one of the bridesmen and maids (as the custom is here) went up to the bride, took off the veil and wreath, and put on a jaunty cap, making a very nice speech that "she is no longer young *frau*, but wife become," and wishing all sorts of good and noble wishes.

After dessert, the happy pair were to go to their temporary home, one of their vineyards, where they are to pass two weeks. They found their coachman was in a drunken sleep, and it took long to arouse him; so, they were an hour late, and after the first *adieus*, came back and took ices and coffee. Then there came a thunder storm; but finally, they started, and then the rest danced out the bride's wreath and the groom's bouquet to see who would be the next bride and groom. After that, somebody had the temerity to propose a dance; so, the pastor left and the mamma and the sisters retired to the next room, and the others danced till eleven, when we were all glad to go home.

Tharant, June 6, 1873.
I forgot; I have a pleasant piece of news for you. Sorge (a brother-in-law) sent especially for me to come in, and when I came, appeared with all his orders on and presented me with one that he had been commanded to give me, together with a certificate of my services in the war. (See note following). I was so surprised and delighted, too; so now you see I have two from the good old emperor, and, if I don't love him forever, whom can I love? I have my photograph taken with them both, and so soon

as they are done shall send you one. I know it's the stupidest vanity, but everybody here insisted so that I did it.

★★★★★★

Berlin, June 14, 1873.

It gives the undersigned Department great pleasure to be able to send to Mrs. Mary Olnhausen of Lexington, North America, the war medal for 1870-71 for non-combatants and also the certificate for the great service which she has rendered the wounded; which (medal and certificate) were granted to her by the supreme cabinet order of December 19 of last year.

Your most honourable body is most obediently requested to prepare the respective Insignia for the lady in question according to agreement.

War Department—Military Medical Department.

(Signature.) (Signature.)

To the Royal High Commissioner of Buildings, Honourable Mr. Sorge, Dresden.

★★★★★★

Tharant, June 8, 1873.

Your letter of the 18th of May came yesterday in the midst of very dirty work; and I was so glad both for the letter and a chance to rest a little, for M. and I were grubbing in the cellars. We are, of course, very busy now preparing for the auction, which comes tomorrow week, and such a pile of useless old things as were brought to light could only be found in a German house. I see more than ever how much sentiment is wasted in this world. Both Sister and her M. would never bring themselves to destroy or even part with anything that had ever had any sentiment for them or anybody dear to them; and see now a most unsentimental American comes and, without one bit of heart in the matter, ruthlessly tears, burns, and destroys the *ganze* thing. M. looks on as if it were a church sacrilege; she won't bring herself to help in the deed, but silently acquiesces. We were all invited to a coffee-party, and as they would not go without me, I had to go against my will. If I were a good mimic, I could make you laugh over it. I never saw so many comical people together. Two sisters, Fraülein von ——, somebody ought to picture them! In the first place two such original styles of homeliness exist *nicht*. One is the energetic sort, head very far back set; talks housekeeping and maids unendlessly; eyes so

190

wide open you don't catch her napping; masterful of everybody, her maid don't crib much from her; talks herself red in the face over the slightest thing, and sees-out like a mad dog if she is a little opposed; knows the whole gossip of every house in town, with the deepest sympathy inquires over one's most tender affairs, and gives advice on all occasions.

The other has alarmingly red cheeks, but otherwise pale; holds her head forward, a *bischen* sunken in such a deprecatory manner, and always acquiesces,—*jah, jah*, going on all the time in a sort of monotone that is a little wearing. Na! you must see that. Evidently they like *beaux*, and they are always adjusting something.

The lady of the house, too, is a character. She is constantly forgetting names, and gets hopelessly confused; and her two daughters are always trying to put her right, which, of course, always goes wrong. Those coffees are, anyway, not the most agreeable things; and then one is expected to eat such a succession of fatty sweets that one must have dyspepsia for a week afterwards. I know I was just glad when seven o'clock came and we could go home.

The holidays lasted three days; on the third, one of those sisters (the submissive one) came out from Dresden in the evening train with her maid; when in the depot a drunken student seized her, and another her maid, and compelled them to dance. Imagine the scene, this dignified gentle woman, protesting all the while, being wheeled around in such an undignified manner, and the whole crowd looking on and enjoying it.

Tharant, July 16, 1873.

The 14th I went in to Thode's (her banker), and he telegraphed a second time for the *Marathon*, 31st; and this morning I have the answer that my berth is engaged; so now it's about certain I shall sail in that. I shall allow about a week for the journey to Liverpool, as I want to stop a day in Hamburg, and, if possible, see a little of at least one city in England. London is out of the question. I shall take the shortest and cheapest route; and, anyway, now I am certain of going home, I shall not enjoy much that I see. It is a very exciting time with me now. The parting from my friends here is very hard, and yet the desire to see you all quite deadens the pain.

191

Chapter 11

The "wonderful aunt from America" might have remained many years on the other side of the Atlantic and have found an unflagging welcome in the households of her late husband's kin. As her later letters make clear, however, she was eager to get home; not simply because of a natural wish to see her own people, but also and chiefly because long-continued idleness had become irksome to her. Her first thought, therefore, after recovering from the excitement of the homecoming, was to find some position where she might be usefully employed and might at the same time earn her own living. Independence, both in purse and in dwelling-place, was essential to her happiness.

At any time during the remaining thirty years of her life, shelter and leisure in the homes of her many relatives would gladly have been hers; but, however welcome she might be, such a life was practically impossible to her. She could scarcely exist in an ordinary household. She must have her own gods about her, must keep her own house—however tiny—in her own Bohemian way. Possessing hosts of friends, she must be able to have them always about her and to entertain them with "picnics" of her own devising. She must be free to go about visiting, to the theatre, upon expeditions of all kinds without question except of her own good sense, and without responsibility except to her own high breeding.

Above all, she hated the thought of dependence upon others for her daily bread. So, to the very end of her long life she earned that bread herself, (see note following); and even after her eightieth year, when the fact of her living by herself was a source of great anxiety to her friends, she could not be persuaded to give up the independence which, surrounded by her "traps," she so much enjoyed in her hospitable quarters in the Grundmann Studios.

★★★★★★

In 1888, through the exertions of Hon. E. D. Hayden, M. C. from Massachusetts, she was given, by vote of the Congress, a pension of twelve dollars a month.

★★★★★★

About the time of her return from Europe, a Training School for Nurses, affiliated with the Massachusetts General Hospital, in Boston, was established, and to Mrs. von Olnhausen was offered the position of superintendent.

★★★★★★

From the Seventeenth Annual Report of Trustees of the Massachusetts General Hospital (1883), p. 6: "This Institution began in 1873 with six pupils, who were allowed to take charge of two wards as an experiment. It increased steadily till 1877, when the nursing of the whole Hospital was placed in its charge. At the present time (1883) the Training School consists of forty-two pupils, twelve head nurses, a night superintendent, and the superintendent of the whole school,—all these being under the supervision of a Board of Directors."

★★★★★★

The writer saw much of her at that time, and although he was but a lad, remembers well her cheeriness and breeziness, her kind word to every patient, her untiring efforts to keep them buoyed up and entertained. That scrupulous attention to cleanliness, too, and that wonderful skill in the treatment of wounds which had distinguished her army service, were again conspicuous. But, boy as he was, he could see that his aunt had not the qualifications essential for the post which, with unflagging zeal, she was trying so enthusiastically to fill. She was not systematic, and a hospital must be run as if by clockwork. She was not autocratic, and women seeking to be trained as nurses need the firm and steady hand of high authority. She was absolutely blunt and always ready to speak her mind, and her experimental position called for the utmost tact and discretion.

She was by nature a person of violent likes and dislikes, and her situation forbade the slightest exhibition of favouritism. Moreover, wide and wonderful as her experience had been, it had not given her a thorough training in the principles of nursing, and her mind had not been steadied and disciplined by that higher education which, had she been born fifty years later, she undoubtedly would eagerly have sought. It is not to be wondered at, therefore, that she did not succeed in a position demanding qualities which by nature and by education were not hers. After a year or two at the Training School it became inevitable that she should resign.

Her next position, taken only temporarily, was as matron of a small home for intemperate women in New York City. Thence she went to Staten Island as superintendent of a maternity asylum which had been established, by private charity, in a beautiful spot on the hills of the interior. Two large estates, each with extensive grounds, had been thrown into one; in the two mansion houses and in a number of cottages were sheltered several hundred women and their children; and the work there carried on of rescue, of reform, of provision for the future of the children was most beneficent.

Here was an occupation suited exactly to Mary von Olnhausen's temperament. Her vigour and activity found full scope in the care of the many buildings and the oversight of their varied and ever-changing inmates; her unfailing cheerfulness and her downrightness of speech were excellent tonics for the unfortunate women with whom she had to deal; best of all, her unbounded sympathy and faith in human nature surrounded those unhappy beings with an atmosphere essential to the process of their regeneration.

Living wholly with and for her charges, she had at once to be housekeeper, head nurse, *confidante*, steward, adviser. One hour she must devise means of keeping secluded some erring member of society, the next she must teach the cooks how to prepare some wholesome dish for the sick, the next she must advise with the trustees in regard to the placing of a new lot of children. This woman must be reasoned with, that scolded, the third taught to sew.

Learning, one day, that a murderously drunken husband is pounding at the door, she drops his frantic wife and children, who had sought refuge with her, out of a window, pilots them through the woods, herself drives them to a place of safety, and returns to tell bold lies to the man thus circumvented. Another day she must plan a campaign for the capture of a madman escaped from an asylum and roaming over her grounds threatening death to everyone. These but faintly indicate the kind of problems that were always meeting her. Night and day, she must be everywhere, must think of everything, must be the motive force and the guiding hand in this large and difficult establishment.

This excellent haven of refuge, however, had been built up almost solely by the exertions of a splendid, indomitable woman possessed of large means and of marked executive ability. She was aggressive and positive; Mrs. von Olnhausen, also and equally, was positive, aggressive, and out spoken. Both loved the work, and each was confident that hers was the only way in which it should be carried on. It was impossible, therefore, that sooner or later there should not be wide and irreconcilable differences of opinion between this organiser of the charity and the woman whom she had placed in charge of it.

After several years of happy and useful work, the time came when the position held by Mrs. von Olnhausen was no longer tenable; and, with a sorrowful heart, she gave it up. Then, rather than be dependent, she accepted the position of housekeeper with a family not far from Boston.

Meanwhile the Centennial Exposition, at Philadelphia, had aroused us Americans to an appreciation of artistic decoration; and many women had become fired with a desire to substitute for the "tidies" and "antimacassars" of an earlier generation really beautiful and artistic pieces of embroidery. Although it was many years since she had been a designer of fabrics at Manchester, Mary von Olnhausen had not lost her facility of hand or of invention.

Always skilful with her needle, her residence among German women had taught her many new secrets of the embroiderer's art; and her love and deep knowledge of nature made it possible for her to use flowers, leaves, and vines, in designing, with an artistic freedom that was a revelation to those whose ideas had been bounded by the conventional abominations of the "stamped" pattern. Establishing herself, then, as a designer and maker of embroideries, she soon found that this was indeed her vocation, and that thus she might realise her wish to gain a livelihood without losing the independence essential to her happiness.

For more than twenty years Mrs. von Olnhausen continued to follow this congenial work of producing beautiful designs and exquisite embroideries and of teaching others how to make them. Her imagination seemed never to fail her, her fingers lost none of their cunning, and, most extraordinary of all, her eyes served her faithfully, under the tremendous strain placed upon them, up to the very end. All day, and far into the night sometimes, she would sit over her designing, her swift fingers fashioning beautiful curves and flower and leaf forms, without any aid from instruments, and yet the complicated lines resolving themselves at last into a well thought out design of that freely conventional order which is of the highest degree of decorative art.

Or one would find her sitting with a book propped before her, reading attentively, while her fingers wove intricate stitches of embroidery. Always busy, she nevertheless read an astonishing number of books—in English, French, and German—and reached an opinion concerning them that was of definite value. More than this, she found time to go frequently to the theatre and to hear much good music,— her many friends being only too glad to invite so vivacious and appreciative a companion.

Her room was always open to, and was generally crowded with those hosts of friends; and her greatest delight was to prepare for them with her own hands a little "feast," cooked as only she could cook. However, few the dishes and however primitive the table furnishings, these "picnics" were made veritable banquets by her wit and gayety.

Living at the "Pavilion," opposite King's Chapel, until that house was pulled down, she had rooms subsequently in various places in Boston, until, on the conversion of the Winslow Skating Rink into the Grundmann Studios, she established herself there, and there remained, when in town, almost to the end. Her residence in Boston was not, however, continuous.

It was broken by visits of longer or shorter duration to the houses of her sisters; and several summers were spent in Annisquam, that quaint village of Cape Ann, where she took a building in which sail-boats had formerly been constructed, and, with a few boards and bright chintzes, converted it into a charming cottage. Its loft was divided into several rooms, and from the sitting-room one stepped out upon a balcony actually overhanging the waters of the bay; its first floor was made into a huge kitchen-dining-room, with wide double doors framing the panorama of the Squam River, and with the sea, at high tide, splashing and murmuring under its very floor.

One winter was spent with a cousin in Warner, New Hampshire; a part of another was passed at Shackelford Island,—that long sand-bar off Morehead City where Mrs. von Olnhausen had enjoyed so many pleasant hours during the Civil War; and once more, after a visit to the Columbian Exposition and to relatives in St. Louis, she went to take care of that brother to whom twice before, on the Illinois prairie, she had given such efficient help.

This time, however, he was living on the plains of South Dakota, and alone. His children, now married, were more or less widely scattered; he himself was obliged to be much away; the lake on whose shores he had established himself had, as is so often the case in that semi-arid region, vanished; and with it had gone the hundred neighbours whom this rare sheet of water had originally attracted thither. Not far off, too, was a reservation for Indians, of whom Mrs. von Olnhausen seems to have stood in a fear most unusual with her. Many a long day and gruesome evening, therefore, did she pass sitting at the door of that Dakota house, the vast prairie, broken only by the deserted houses, stretching limitlessly before her, even the beloved nature-sounds transformed, to her excited imagination, into Indian footsteps,—watching for her brother to return.

The easy care of the house was but a meagre outlet for such energy as hers; the solitude of the prairie was a contrast too sharp for one who had lived so long in a city and amid a crowd of friends.

From this last Western visit, she came back what, in spite of her seventy-five years, she had not before been,—an aged woman. Her activities, her innocent pleasure-seeking, her work for others did not cease; but the marvellous buoyancy of what had seemed eternal youth in her was gone.

Mary von Olnhausen was so modest, she was so much more ready to hear the stories of others than to tell her own, that few realised what a heroine of romance this little teacher of embroidery had been. The much-heralded coming of Prince Henry of Prussia to this country happened, however, to call the attention of the newspapers to her whom they named "The Little Madam of the Iron Cross," and she was thereafter much exploited. From Maine to California the story of her life was carried; she became the fashion; her room was crowded by persons with and without introductions; orders for embroideries poured in upon her, and she existed during the last months of her lifetime in a whirl of excitement that could not but prove too trying for a woman of her years.

On the day of the prince's coming, the German women who were received by him insisted that she should accompany them. Entering the room where the ladies were awaiting him, the *Kaiser's* brother immediately noticed the Iron Cross which she wore, and, ignoring formality, grasped her hand and spoke to her in German. Finding that she failed to understand him, he then addressed her in English, inquired about her services, and promised that a duplicate of the lost "Cross of Merit" should be sent to her. The newspapers made much of this recognition of her; but her own simple account given in a letter to a friend in North Carolina, who had sent her some galax leaves, is the best:—

197

The leaves are most beautiful. I have never seen any handsomer. They came the day I went to see the prince, but I did not take him any, and have regretted since that I did not; but it was so formidable, and I am such a fool, I only wanted it over. He was most gracious, and not at all formidable; shook my hand twice, just as any other *feller* would. I am glad I had the courage now to go, especially on account of the younger nieces and nephews, who were so anxious for me to do so. They have been making a great fuss in the papers; of course, it's all exaggerated. Really, the whole thing was what anyone would have done much better than I did, only I had the luck. How splendidly you would have carried out the meeting and handshaking! I forgot to bow low or to address him with any title; so stupid!

It has been a hard winter for me, in the hospital and at home, and I am away behind in my finances; but if the orders come as thick as they have this last week, I shall soon be independent. Nothing like being the *fad* for a while. I've waited forty years, and now, when I'm so old, it comes all at once. It has been a bad winter here, they say. So far, I've not been out, except to ride; but I have some engagements for this week, so shall have to trot around, besides working night and day, for a while. How I long for the spring and the birds and frogs! You have had them long ago, I suppose.

This is one of the last letters that she wrote. Going soon afterwards to Lexington for a visit, she was seized with apoplexy, and, without suffering or return of consciousness, passed away on the twelfth day of April, 1902. Two days later she was taken to Mount Auburn Chapel; a flag was pinned upon her breast by the Army Nurses Association; a larger flag was twined among the beautiful flowers upon her coffin; fitting words of memorial were spoken by the Rev. Carlton A. Staples, minister of the First Church in Lexington,—the church where, as a girl, she had come every Sunday with her family; and she was put to rest beside the dear husband from whom she had been parted so many years before.

The life of which these letters give but inadequate glimpses was interesting above all because it was so intensely human. Its virtues were common virtues, its shortcomings were common faults; but both were intensified by the extraordinary vigour, by the unique personality of Mary von Olnhausen. Her very presence breathed an abounding vitality; and it was that, doubtless, almost as much as her skill in nursing, which revived and stimulated into health again her many patients. She gloried in making men live whose hurts had been pronounced incurable. Between her, the healer, and them, the suffering, there was, for the time, a human bond as close as between members of one family. For that reason, she could seldom perceive the faults or unworthiness of any man who had been a patient in her hands. But, as she liked with intensity, so she hated intensely; and there was often as much of unreason in the one attitude as in the other.

It is probable, therefore, that some of the dangers and discomforts which she experienced were due not wholly to others, but, in a measure, to herself. For she could not wheedle, she would not placate, and she often placed dependence upon the untrue, while distrusting the true friend. Her nature was so open, however, that it is easy to correct, as men of science do, for the personal equation in her letters, and to see, as she saw, the seamy side of battles, to learn, as she learned, how quickly and surely war brings to the front all the evil, hideous, barbarous passions of mankind. Many of her experiences, however, were too revolting to be placed upon a printed page, many of her discomforts were too intimately associated with individuals for it to be wise to publish them.

Nevertheless, these suppressions, the still greater pruning of the letters through the omission of personal references and of pages interesting only to her friends, have not been sufficient to hide the rare character of Mary von Olnhausen, to spoil the value of the varied pictures which she draws. Of an extraordinary physique, she was not only ready, she was anxious, to expend that vigorous health in service of the most exacting kind. Loving intensely and hating fiercely, she scorned to make selfish use of the love of others, refused ever to feed hate with innuendo. Generous to a fault, she would give her last cent to relieve suffering, would share her remaining crust with anyone asking hospitality.

Different from other women, but never conspicuous; Bohemian, but careful of the prejudices of others; in dependent, but not in the least self-assertive; free of language, but hating everything coarse; exaggerated in statement, but always scrupulous as to the underlying truth; bold of speech, but tender of heart; often deceived by human beings, but never losing her sublime trust in human nature; of no particular creed, but with abiding faith in God,—she exhibited in her eighty-fourth year, as in youth and in middle age, the beautiful and endearing qualities of childhood, she showed the trust, the purity, the glad exuberance of a little girl.

Her life, in a way, anticipated the development of the nineteenth century. Not till the close of that hundred years did men learn really to love and to understand nature; she possessed that love and knowledge as a girl. Not till well after the middle of that century did women free themselves from the thrall of Biblical and Puritan tradition; she, as a young woman, quietly and modestly defied conventions, and lived, worked, and thought freely, as do men.

The chief triumph of the nineteenth century has been in its understanding of true philanthropy, in its putting into actual practice, on a large and general scale, the Golden Rule. Mary von Olnhausen early found her happiness in living, in suffering, in encountering hardships for the sake of others. She was too human to be a saint, of too intense a vitality to be thoroughly well balanced; but she was what the world most needs,—an unflagging, unselfish, optimistic moral force.

Appendix A

When this volume was in press certain documents came to light which show Baron von Olnhausen to have been a schoolboy in Oehringen, Württemberg, in 1823-24, a pupil at the Royal Bavarian School at Augsburg in 1825 and 1826, a candidate in Philosophy at the University of Munich in 1827 and 1828, and a chemist at Prague in 1833. From other sources, it has been learned that in 1840 he was studying at Edinburgh University.

Excerpts, in literal translation, from some of the documents follow:—

Extract from the opinions relative to the pupils of the fourth Gymnasium class, school-year 1824/25.

von Ohlnhausen Gustav, pupil of the fourth Gymnasium class, son of a merchant, born at Zwickau, Kingdom of Saxony, age 16 years 7 months, (he must have been born, therefore, in February, 1809), is recommended by his bearing, modesty and mental capacity, which are further enhanced by the gift of a pleasant speech; and whose progress in religion is good, in mathematics excellent.

General Qualifying Remarks.

Capabilities—great.

Industry—very great, in mathematics excellent, almost untiring.

Conduct—excellent.

Progress—very good. Twelfth among 45 fellow students.

Augsburg, September 7, 1825.

★★★★★★

In the Lyceum class of the Royal Bavarian Institution of Learning here, *Mr. Gustav von Olnhausen,* from Zwickau, in the Kingdom of Saxony, has deserved, in the first semester of the school year 1825/26, in the studies of the first year course of philosophy and general sciences, being endowed with many mental gifts, the following record:—

Subject	Industry	Progress
Universal History	Excellent	Excellent
Latin Literature	"	Very good
Greek Literature	"	" "
Logic	Very good	" "
Metaphysics	" "	Excellent
Religion	Excellent	"
Algebra	Untiring	"
Trigonometry	"	"

His mental development was exemplary.
This is attested by the undersigned authorities

(Signatures.)

Augsburg, August 20, 1826.

******

(*Certificate*) That the Candidate in Philosophy, Mr. Gustav von Olnhausen, from Oehringen, in the Kingdom of Württemberg, has been at the University here for purposes of study from November 18, 1826, up to date, during this time has observed a faultless conduct in conformity with the requirements, and has not committed any wrong with regard to proscribed societies. This is attested, at his desire, at his departure from this University.

Munich, August 14, 1828.

Royal University Rector
Dr. J. Doellinger.

******

Passport

Mr. Gustav Adolph von Olnhausen, who at present is in Prague, as chemist, born here in 1809, and against whose stay in Prague there is no objection here, since, more particularly, there is no claim for military service,—such facts are hereby certified for his assistance.

Zwickau in the Kingdom of Saxony
City Council

Friedrich Wilhelm Meyer.

18th December, 1833.

Appendix B

In the recently published *Life and Correspondence of Henry Ingersoll Bowditch* (by his son, Vincent Y. Bowditch, Houghton, Mifflin & Co., 1902) appears the following letter (vol. ii.):

To Mrs. George L. Stearns.

May 9, 1887.

Dear Mrs. Stearns,—I forgot to leave with you the riddle, (inserted below paragraph) found in a book of autographs made chiefly between the years 1610 and 1630. The riddle has the date of 1742, and is signed by one Fulda, at that time the possessor of the precious heirlooms of the family Von Olnhausen; and which had been carefully kept and transmitted to sons of that name for one hundred and thirty-two years. The Von Olnhausens dated their origin from a gallant Crusader, Heinrich Olnhausen, who in 1388 had been made "Knight of the Golden Spur" at Jerusalem.

★★★★★★

AMORES
6. Sex fuge,
5. Quinque tene,
4. Quatuor fac,
Reliqua (RES) tibi sequentur.

★★★★★★

The autographs collected by one of his descendants (an earnest student, between 1610 and 1630) of all the great personages (nobility with their illuminated coats of arms, professors of many universities, pastors of churches, great physicians, and lettered young companions) were in two volumes, and by marriage had come into Fulda's hands. He, with a true instinct, felt that they ought to be in the hands of his young relative, the male descendant of the Von Olnhausens. Therefore in 1742 he transferred them to John Frederick Olnhausen, telling him that he hoped that these precious relics of the good youth of 1610 would stimulate his loving descendants to behave as heroically as his predecessors had done, and he gave the enclosed riddle, which as I have before stated I forgot to leave.

To finish my story, I ought to tell you how they came into my possession. Some few years before the war of the rebel lion, a tall, middle-aged German came into my study, evidently very ill, I saw at a glance. There was intellect and great suffering seen in his face, but there was a serenity of manner and quietness of speech which charmed me. I soon found that he was hopelessly ill; his wife, an American woman, flitted around him, watching tenderly every word that fell from him. It was evident that they were poor.

I advised him to enter a hospital, and I visited him as a friend several times before he died. I found that he was a patriot obliged to leave Germany, and had sought this country, devoted as he thought to freedom, and shocked he had been to find how rampant slavery was here. Just before death he willed to me his Schiller cup, from which he had drunk Rhenish wine from the time of student life on the anniversary of the poet's birth. He had brought the autograph books here, he being the last male descendant of his race.

His wife soon after his death left the books with me for safe-keeping, when she entered as a nurse the Northern hospital. After serving till the end of the war, she went to Germany and offered herself, and was accepted, as a nurse in the Franco-Prussian War. By a strange coincidence, among her first patients was one named Olnhausen. He was of the family of her husband. She subsequently lived there some weeks (years), and then returned to America.

Excuse me for this lengthy story. When I fall upon the history of a really excellent German patient or friend I find much to interest me, and my pen flows on freely.

I remain very sincerely yours,

Henry I. Bowditch.

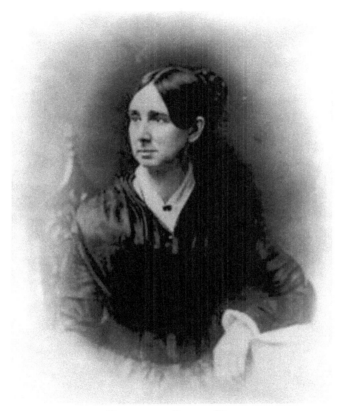

Dorothea Lynde Dix

Dorothea L. Dix

By L. P. Brockett

Among all the women who devoted themselves with untiring energy, and gave talents of the highest order to the work of caring for our soldiers during the war, the name of Dorothea L. Dix will always take the first rank, and history will undoubtedly preserve it long after all others have sunk into oblivion. This her extraordinary and exceptional official position will secure. Others have doubtless done as excellent a work, and earned a praise equal to her own, but her relations to the government will insure her historical mention and remembrance, while none will doubt the sincerity of her patriotism, or the faithfulness of her devotion.

Dorothea L. Dix is a native of Worcester, Mass. Her father was a physician, who died while she was as yet young, leaving her almost without pecuniary resources.

Soon after this event, she proceeded to Boston, where she opened a select school for young ladies, from the income of which she was enabled to draw a comfortable support.

One day during her residence in Boston, while passing along a street, she accidentally overheard two gentlemen, who were walking before her, conversing about the state prison at Charlestown, and expressing their sorrow at the neglected condition of the convicts. They were undoubtedly of that class of philanthropists who believe that no man, however vile, is *all* bad, but, though sunk into the lowest depths of vice, has yet in his soul some white spot which the taint has not reached, but which some kind hand may reach, and some kind heart may touch.

Be that as it may, their remarks found an answering chord in the heart of Miss Dix. She was powerfully affected and impressed, so much so, that she obtained no rest until she had herself visited the prison, and learned that in what she had heard there was no exaggeration. She found great suffering, and great need of reform.

Energetic of character, and kindly of heart, she at once lent herself to the work of elevating and instructing the degraded and suffering classes she found there, and becoming deeply interested in the welfare of these unfortunates, she continued to employ herself in labours pertaining to this field of reform, until the year 1834.

At that time, her health becoming greatly impaired, she gave up her school and embarked for Europe. Shortly before this period, she had inherited from a relative sufficient property to render her independent of daily exertion for support, and to enable her to carry out any plans of charitable work which she should form. Like all persons firmly fixed in an idea which commends itself alike to the judgment and the impulses, she was very tenacious of her opinions relating to it, and impatient of opposition. It is said that from this cause, she did not always meet the respect and attention which the important objects to which she was devoting her life would seem to merit. That she found friends and helpers however at home and abroad, is undoubtedly true.

She remained abroad until the year 1837, when returning to her native country she devoted herself to the investigation of the condition of paupers, lunatics and prisoners. In this work, she was warmly aided and encouraged by her friend and pastor the Rev. Dr. Channing, of whose children she had been governess, as well as by many other persons whose hearts beat a chord responsive to that long since awakened in her own.

Since 1841 until the breaking out of the late war, Miss Dix devoted herself to the great work which she accepted as the special mission of her life. In pursuance of it, she, during that time, is said to have visited every State of the Union east of the Rocky Mountains, examining prisons, poor-houses, lunatic asylums, and endeavouring to persuade legislatures and influential individuals to take measures for the relief of the poor and wretched.

Her exertions contributed greatly to the foundation of State lunatic asylums in Rhode Island, Pennsylvania, New York, Indiana, Illinois, Louisiana and North Carolina. She presented a memorial to Congress during the Session of 1848-9, asking an appropriation of five hundred thousand acres of the public lands to endow hospitals for the indigent insane.

This measure failed, but, not discouraged, she renewed the appeal in 1850 asking for ten millions of acres. The Committee of the House to whom the memorial was referred, made a favourable report, and a bill such as she asked for passed the House, but failed in the Senate for want of time. In April, 1854, however, her unwearied exertions were rewarded by the passage of a bill by both houses, appropriating ten millions of acres to the several States for the relief of the indigent insane. But this bill was vetoed by President Pierce, chiefly on the ground that the General Government had no constitutional power to make such appropriations.

Miss Dix was thus unexpectedly checked and deeply disappointed in the immediate accomplishment of this branch of the great work of benevolence to which she had more particularly devoted herself.

From that time, she seems to have given herself, with added zeal, to her labours for the insane. This class so helpless, and so innocently suffering, seem to have always been, and more particularly during the later years of her work, peculiarly the object of her sympathies and labours. In the prosecution of these labours she made another voyage to Europe in 1858 or '59, and continued to pursue them with indefatigable zeal and devotion.

The labours of Miss Dix for the insane were continued without intermission until the occurrence of those startling events which at once turned into other and new channels nearly all the industries and philanthropies of our nation. With many a premonition, and many a muttering of the coming storm, unheeded, our people, inured to peace, continued unappalled in their quiet pursuits. But while the actual commencement of active hostilities called thousands of men to arms, from the monotony of mechanical, agricultural and commercial pursuits and the professions, it changed as well the thoughts and avocations of those who were not to enter the ranks of the military.

And not to men alone did these changes come. Not they alone were filled with a new fire of patriotism, and a quickened devotion to the interests of our nation. Scarcely had the ear ceased thrilling with the tidings that our country was indeed the theatre of civil war, when women as well as men began to inquire if there were not for them some part to be played in this great drama.

Almost, if not quite the first among these was Miss Dix. Self-reliant, accustomed to rapid and independent action, conscious of her ability for usefulness, with her to resolve was to act. Scarcely had the first regiments gone forward to the defence of our menaced capital, when she followed, full of a patriotic desire to *offer* to her country whatever service a woman could perform in this hour of its need, and determined that it should be given.

She passed through Baltimore shortly after that fair city had covered itself with the indelible disgrace of the 16th of April, 1861, and on her arrival at Washington, the first labour she offered on her country's altar, was the nursing of some wounded soldiers, victims of the Baltimore mob. Thus, was she earliest in the field.

Washington became a great camp. Everyone was willing, nay anxious, to be useful and employed. Military hospitals were hastily organised. There were many sick, but few skilful nurses. The opening of the rebellion had not found the government, nor the loyal people prepared for it. All was confusion, want of discipline, and disorder. Organising minds, persons of executive ability, *leaders*, were wanted.

The services of women could be made available in the hospitals. They were needed as nurses, but it was equally necessary that someone should decide upon their qualifications for the task, and direct their efforts.

Miss Dix was present in Washington. Her ability, long experience in public institutions and high character were well known. Scores of persons of influence, from all parts of the country, could vouch for her, and she had already offered her services to the authorities for any work in which they could be made available.

Her selection for the important post of Superintendent of Female Nurses, by Secretary Cameron, then at the head of the War Department, on the 10th of June, 1861, commanded universal approbation.

This at once opened for her a wide and most important field of duty and labour. Except hospital matrons, (in many instances she appointed these also), all women regularly employed in the hospitals, and entitled to pay from the Government, were appointed by her. An examination of the qualifications of each applicant was made. A woman must be mature in years, plain almost to homeliness in dress, and by no means liberally endowed with personal attractions, if she hoped to meet the approval of Miss Dix. Good health and an unexceptionable moral character were always insisted on.

As the war progressed, the applications were numerous, and the need of this kind of service great, but the rigid scrutiny first adopted by Miss Dix continued, and many were rejected who did not in all respects possess the qualifications which she had fixed as her standard. Some of these women, who in other branches of the service, and under other auspices, became eminently useful, were rejected on account of their youth while some, alas! were received, who afterwards proved themselves quite unfit for the position, and a disgrace to their sex.

But in these matters no blame can attach to Miss Dix. In the first instance, she acted no doubt from the dictates of a sound and mature judgment; and in the last was often deceived by false testimonials, by a specious appearance, or by applicants who, innocent at the time, were not proof against the temptations and allurements of a position which all must admit to be peculiarly exposed and unsafe.

Besides the appointment of nurses, the position of Miss Dix imposed upon her numerous and onerous duties. She visited hospitals, far and near, inquiring into the wants of their occupants, in all cases where possible, supplementing the government stores by those with which she was always supplied by private benevolence, or from public sources; she adjusted disputes, and settled difficulties in which her nurses were concerned; and in every way showed her true and untiring devotion to her country, and its suffering defenders.

She undertook long journeys by land and by water, and seemed ubiquitous, for she was seldom missed from her office in Washington, yet was often seen elsewhere, and always bent upon the same fixed and earnest purpose. We cannot, perhaps, better describe the personal appearance of Miss Dix, and give an idea of her varied duties and many sacrifices, than by transcribing the following extract from the printed correspondence of a lady, herself an active and most efficient labourer in the same general field of effort, and holding an important position in the North-western Sanitary Commission.

It was Sunday morning when we arrived in Washington, and as the Sanitary Commission held no meeting that day, we decided after breakfast to pay a visit to Miss Dix.

We fortunately found the good lady at home, but just ready to start for the hospitals. She is slight and delicate looking, and seems physically inadequate to the work she is engaged in. In her youth she must have possessed considerable beauty, and she is still very comely, with a soft and musical voice, graceful figure, and very winning manners. Secretary Cameron vested her with sole power to appoint female nurses in the hospitals. Secretary Stanton, on succeeding him ratified the appointment, and she has installed several hundreds of nurses in this noble work—all of them Protestants, and middle-aged. Miss Dix's whole soul is in this work.

She rents two large houses, which are depots for sanitary supplies sent to her care, and houses of rest and refreshment for nurses and convalescent soldiers, employs two secretaries, owns ambulances and keeps them busily employed, prints and distributes circulars, goes hither and thither from one remote point to another in her visitations of hospitals,—and pays all the expenses incurred from her private purse. Her fortune, time and strength are laid on the altar of the country in this hour of trial. Unfortunately, many of the surgeons in the hospitals do not work harmoniously with Miss Dix. They are jealous of her power, impatient of her authority, find fault with her nurses, and accuse her of being arbitrary, opinionated, severe and capricious. Many to rid themselves of her entirely, have obtained permission of Surgeon-General Hammond to employ Sisters of Charity in their hospitals, a proceeding not to Miss Dix's liking. Knowing by observation that many of the surgeons are wholly unfit for their office, that too often they fail to bring skill, morality, or humanity to their work, we could easily understand how this single-hearted, devoted, tireless friend of the sick and wounded soldier would come in collision with these laggards, and we liked her none the less for it.

Though Miss Dix received no salary, devoting to the work her time and labours without remuneration, a large amount of supplies were placed in her hands, both by the Government and from private sources, which she was always ready to dispense with judgment and caution, it is true, but with a pleasant earnestness alike grateful to the recipient of the kindness, or to the agent who acted in her stead in this work of mercy.

It was perhaps unfortunate for Miss Dix that at the time when she received her appointment it was so unprecedented, and the entire service was still in such a chaotic state, that it was simply impossible to define her duties or her authority. As, therefore, no plan of action or rules were adopted, she was forced to abide exclusively by her own ideas of need and authority. In a letter to the writer, from an official source, her position and the changes that became necessary are thus explained:

The appointment of nurses was regulated by her ideas of their prospective usefulness, good moral character being an absolute prerequisite. This absence of system, and independence of action, worked so very unsatisfactorily, that in October, 1863, a

General Order was issued placing the assignment, or employment of female nurses, exclusively under control of Medical Officers, and limiting the superintendency to a 'certificate of approval,' without which no woman nurse could be employed, except by order of the Surgeon-General. This materially reduced the number of appointments, secured the muster and pay of those in service, and established discipline and order.

The following is the General Order above alluded to.

General Orders, No. 351.
War Department, Adjutant-General's Office,
Washington, October 29, 1863.

The employment of women nurses in the United States General Hospitals will in future be strictly governed by the following rules:

1. Persons approved by Miss Dix, or her authorised agents, will receive from her, or them, "certificates of approval," which must be countersigned by Medical Directors upon their assignment to duty as nurses within their Departments.

2. Assignments of "women nurses" to duty in General Hospitals will only be made upon application by the Surgeons in charge, through Medical Directors, to Miss Dix or her agents, for the number they require, not exceeding one to every thirty beds.

3. No females, except Hospital Matrons, will be. employed in General Hospitals, or, after December 31, 1863, born upon the Muster and Pay Rolls, without such certificates of approval and regular assignment, unless specially appointed by the Surgeon-General.

4. Women nurses, while on duty in General Hospitals, are under the exclusive control of the senior medical officer, who will direct their several duties, and may be discharged by him when considered supernumerary, or for incompetency, insubordination, or violation of his orders. Such discharge, with the reasons therefor, being endorsed upon the certificate, will be at once returned to Miss Dix.

By order of the Secretary of War:

E. D. Townsend,
Assistant Adjutant-General.

Official:

By this Order the authority of Miss Dix was better defined, but she continued to labour under the same difficulty which had from the first clogged her efforts. Authority had been bestowed upon her, but not the power to enforce obedience. There was no penalty for disobedience, and persons disaffected, forgetful, or idle, might refuse or neglect to obey with impunity. It will at once be seen that this fact must have resulted disastrously upon her efforts. She doubtless had enemies, (as who has not?), and some were jealous of the power and prominence of her position, while many might even feel unwilling, under any circumstances, to acknowledge, and yield to the authority of a woman.

Added to this she had, in some cases, and probably without any fault on her part, failed to secure the confidence and respect of the surgeons in charge of hospitals. In these facts lay the sources of trials, discouragements, and difficulties, all to be met, struggled with, and, if possible, triumphed over by a woman, standing quite alone in a most responsible, laborious, and exceptional position. It indeed seems most wonderful—almost miraculous—that under such circumstances, such a vast amount of good was accomplished. Had she not accomplished half so much, she still would richly have deserved that highest of plaudits—Well done good and faithful servant!

Miss Dix has one remarkable peculiarity—undoubtedly remarkable in one of her sex which is said, and with truth—to possess great approbativeness. She does not apparently desire fame, she does not enjoy being talked about, even in praise. The approval of her own conscience, the consciousness of performing an unique and useful work, seems quite to suffice her. Few women are so self-reliant, self-sustained, self-centred. And in saying this we but echo the sentiments, if not the words, of an eminent divine who, like herself, was during the whole war devoted to a work similar in its purpose, and alike responsible and arduous.

> She (Miss Dix) is a lady who likes to do things and not have them talked about. She is freer from the love of public reputation than any woman I know. Then her plans are so strictly her own, and always so wholly controlled by her own individual genius and power, that they cannot well be participated in by others, and not much understood.
>
> Miss Dix, I suspect, was as early *in*, as long employed, and as self-sacrificing as any woman who offered her services to the country. She gave herself—body, soul and substance—to the good

work. I wish we had any record of her work, but we have not. I should not dare to speak for her—about her work—except to say that it was extended, patient and persistent beyond anything I know of, dependent on a single-handed effort.

All the testimony goes to show that Miss Dix is a woman endowed with warm feelings and great kindness of heart. It is only those who do not know her, or who have only met her in the conflict of opposing wills, who pronounce her, as some have done, a cold and heartless egotist. Opinionated she may be, because convinced of the general soundness of her ideas, and infallibility of her judgment. If the success of great designs, undertaken and carried through single-handed, furnish warrant for such conviction, she has an undoubted right to hold it.

Her nature is large and generous, yet with no room for narrow grudges, or mean reservations. As a proof of this, her stores were as readily dispensed for the use of a hospital in which the surgeon refused and rejected her nurses, as for those who employed them.

She had the kindest care and oversight over the women she had commissioned. She wished them to embrace every opportunity for the rest and refreshment rendered necessary by their arduous labours. A home for them was established by her in Washington, which at all times opened its doors for then reception, and where she wished them to enjoy that perfect quiet and freedom from care, during their occasional sojourns, which were the best remedies for their weariness and exhaustion of body and soul.

In her more youthful days Miss Dix devoted herself considerably to literary pursuits. She has published several works anonymously— the first of which—*The Garland of Flora*, was published in Boston in 1829. This was succeeded by a number of books for children, among which were *Conversations about Common Things*, *Alice and Ruth*, and *Evening Hours*. She has also published a variety of tracts for prisoners, and has written many memorials to legislative bodies on the subject of the foundation and conducting of Lunatic Asylums.

Miss Dix is gifted with a singularly gentle and persuasive voice, and her manners are said to exert a remarkably controlling influence over the fiercest maniacs.

She is exceedingly quiet and retiring in her deportment, delicate and refined in manner, with great sweetness of expression. She is far from realising the popular idea of the strong-minded woman—loud, boisterous and uncouth, claiming as a right, what might, perhaps, be more readily obtained as a courteous concession. On the contrary, her successes with legislatures and individuals, are obtained by the mildest efforts, which yet lack nothing of persistence and few persons beholding this delicate and retiring woman would imagine they saw in her the champion of the oppressed and suffering classes.

Miss Dix regards her army work but as an episode in her career. She did what she could, and with her devotion of self and high patriotism she would have done no less. She pursued her labours to the end, and her position was not resigned until many months after the close of the war. In fact, she tarried in Washington to finish many an uncompleted task, for some time after her office had been abolished.

When all was done she returned at once to that which she considers her life's work, the amelioration of the condition of the insane.

A large portion of the winter of 1865-6 was devoted to an attempt to induce the Legislature of New York to make better provision for the insane of that State, and to procure, or erect for them, several asylums of small size where a limited number under the care of experienced physicians, might enjoy greater facilities for a cure, and a better prospect of a return to the pursuits and pleasures of life.

Miss Dix now, (1867), resides at Trenton, New Jersey, where she has since the war fixed her abode, travelling thence to the various scenes of her labours. Wherever she may be, and however engaged, we may be assured that her object is the good of some portion of the race, and is worthy of the prayers and blessings of all who love humanity and seek the promotion of its best interests. And to the close of her long and useful life, the thanks, the heartfelt gratitude of every citizen of our common country so deeply indebted to her, and to the many devoted and self-sacrificing women whose efforts she directed, must as assuredly follow her. She belongs now to History, and America may proudly claim her daughter.

LEONAUR

ALSO FROM LEONAUR
AVAILABLE IN SOFTCOVER OR HARDCOVER WITH DUST JACKET

THE WOMAN IN BATTLE *by Loreta Janeta Velazquez*—Soldier, Spy and Secret Service Agent for the Confederacy During the American Civil War.

BOOTS AND SADDLES *by Elizabeth B. Custer*—The experiences of General Custer's Wife on the Western Plains.

FANNIE BEERS' CIVIL WAR *by Fannie A. Beers*—A Confederate Lady's Experiences of Nursing During the Campaigns & Battles of the American Civil War.

LADY SALE'S AFGHANISTAN *by Florentia Sale*—An Indomitable Victorian Lady's Account of the Retreat from Kabul During the First Afghan War.

THE TWO WARS OF MRS DUBERLY *by Frances Isabella Duberly*—An Intrepid Victorian Lady's Experience of the Crimea and Indian Mutiny.

THE REBELLIOUS DUCHESS *by Paul F. S. Dermoncourt*—The Adventures of the Duchess of Berri and Her Attempt to Overthrow French Monarchy.

LADIES OF WATERLOO *by Charlotte A. Eaton, Magdalene de Lancey & Juana Smith*—The Experiences of Three Women During the Campaign of 1815: Waterloo Days by Charlotte A. Eaton, A Week at Waterloo by Magdalene de Lancey & Juana's Story by Juana Smith.

NURSE AND SPY IN THE UNION ARMY *by Sarah Emma Evelyn Edmonds*—During the American Civil War

WIFE NO. 19 *by Ann Eliza Young*—The Life & Ordeals of a Mormon Woman During the 19th Century

DIARY OF A NURSE IN SOUTH AFRICA *by Alice Bron*—With the Dutch-Belgian Red Cross During the Boer War

MARIE ANTOINETTE AND THE DOWNFALL OF ROYALTY *by Imbert de Saint-Amand*—The Queen of France and the French Revolution

THE MEMSAHIB & THE MUTINY *by R. M. Coopland*—An English lady's ordeals in Gwalior and Agra duringthe Indian Mutiny 1857

MY CAPTIVITY AMONG THE SIOUX INDIANS *by Fanny Kelly*—The ordeal of a pioneer woman crossing the Western Plains in 1864

WITH MAXIMILIAN IN MEXICO *by Sara Yorke Stevenson*—A Lady's experience of the French Adventure

AVAILABLE ONLINE AT **www.leonaur.com**
AND FROM ALL GOOD BOOK STORES

07/09

Printed in the USA
CPSIA information can be obtained
at www.ICGtesting.com
LVHW090955261023
762217LV00016B/40